How to Pass the MRCPsych CASC

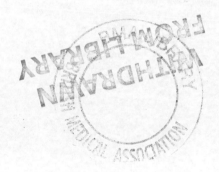

How to Pass the MRCPsych CASC

How to Pass the MRCPsych CASC

Dr Andrew Iles
Specialty Registrar in Forensic Psychiatry, Maudsley Training Scheme, Broadmoor Hospital, UK

Dr Rose Woodall
Specialty Doctor, in Assertive Outreach and General Adult Psychiatry, Birmingham and Solihull Mental Health NHS Foundation Trust, UK

Dr Flavia Leslie
Consultant in General Adult Psychiatry, Berkshire Healthcare NHS Trust, UK

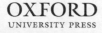

OXFORD
UNIVERSITY PRESS

OXFORD
UNIVERSITY PRESS

Great Clarendon Street, Oxford OX2 6DP

Oxford University Press is a department of the University of Oxford.
It furthers the University's objective of excellence in research, scholarship,
and education by publishing worldwide in

Oxford New York

Auckland Cape Town Dar es Salaam Hong Kong Karachi
Kuala Lumpur Madrid Melbourne Mexico City Nairobi
New Delhi Shanghai Taipei Toronto

With offices in

Argentina Austria Brazil Chile Czech Republic France Greece
Guatemala Hungary Italy Japan Poland Portugal Singapore
South Korea Switzerland Thailand Turkey Ukraine Vietnam

Oxford is a registered trade mark of Oxford University Press
in the UK and in certain other countries

Published in the United States
by Oxford University Press Inc., New York

British Library Cataloguing in Publication Data
Data available

Library of Congress Cataloguing in Publication Data
Data available

Typeset by Glyph International, Bangalore, India
Printed in Great Britain
on acid-free paper by
Ashford Colour Press, Gosport, Hampshire

ISBN 978–0–19–957170–3

10 9 8 7

For our families, for their support

Al and RW

FOREWORD

The Royal College of Psychiatrists have recently changed the way in which the clinical skills of candidates for the MRCPsych are examined. They have introduced the Clinical Assessment of Skills and Competencies (CASC) examination. While it is not possible to learn clinical skills from a book, nevertheless *How to Pass the MRCPsych CASC* will certainly be a great aid to candidates preparing for their CASC examinations.

The authors have the advantage of combining recent experience of sitting the new CASC examination (Dr Andrew Iles and Dr Rose Woodall) with recent experience in being an examiner for this part of the MRCPsych examination (Dr Flavia Leslie). They have brought together their theoretical and practical knowledge to produce an excellent guide for candidates. After explaining the examination and its marking in detail, the book describes important key skills. This is followed by concise details of the major topics that may be examined, including practical skills such as the physical examination of patients, interpretation of the electrocardiogram and resuscitation. Along the way, the authors have included some useful mnemonics, including acronyms such as CANON, DANISH, ITALIC and DICE.

No fewer than ten mock examinations are included in the final part of the book. These provide extremely well thought out learning and practice material. Candidates will benefit enormously by practising taking each of these mock assessments under examination conditions, by forming revision practice groups (with candidates taking it in turn to be the 'patient'), video recording the mock examinations, and assessing these recordings together.

Dr Andrew Iles, Dr Rose Woodall and Dr Flavia Leslie are to be congratulated on having put together such as excellent guide to the CASC. I highly recommend this book.

Professor B.K. Puri,
Hammersmith Hospital and Imperial College London

PREFACE

In 2008 the Royal College of Psychiatrists made a radical change to the way it examines its prospective members. The most significant change is the way in which clinical skills are assessed. The Clinical Assessment of Skills and Competencies (CASC) was introduced. The traditional long case, Patient Management Problems (PMPs), and the observed clinical interview of the old Part 2 examination were all abandoned.

This book has been written by two of the first cohort of trainees to take this new examination and one of the first examiners. It is designed to help other candidates successfully pass the CASC. The approach is unusual in that it does not just contain scripted interviews in response to given scenarios; it combines suggested questions and statements with key facts and evidence from sources such as the National Institute for Clinical Excellence (NICE) and the International Classification of Diseases (ICD-10). This allows the candidate to prepare for a broad range of possible scenarios. The knowledge can then be used to practise the ten mock exams, which include 80 individual stations and 40 pairs of stations, giving the candidate the opportunity to attempt a total of 160 different stations.

As with any professional clinical examination, the CASC requires candidates to demonstrate that they are well-informed and safe clinicians. They must show knowledge of both mental disorders and important physical illnesses, and be able to demonstrate sound management skills. They must also know how to manage risk safely and be able to communicate effectively with patients, carers and colleagues. This book has been written to help you demonstrate these competencies.

We wish you luck.

AI, RW and FL
March 2009

CONTENTS

EXPERT REVIEWERS

General adult
Dr Flavia Leslie BA(Hons), MRCGP, DRCOG, MRCPsych
Consultant Psychiatrist
Berkshire Healthcare NHS Trust

Old Aage
Dr Malcolm B. Liddell MRCPsych, PhD
Consultant Psychiatrist
St Tydfil's Hospital, Merthyr Tydfil

Learning Disability
Dr Val Anness MBChB (Hons), FRCPsych
Consultant Psychiatrist
Hafod Y Wennol, Pontyclun

Child and Adolescent
Dr Tania McGregor MBChB, MRCPsych
Consultant Psychiatrist
South Oxfordshire CAMHS

Substance Misuse
Dr Divya Ganesh Nallur MBBS, MRCPsych, MSc, PG Dip (CBT)
Consultant Psychiatrist
Rhondda Integrated Substance Misuse Team (RISMS), Llwynypia Hospital,

Forensic
Dr Roland M. Jones MBChB, BSc, MSc, MRCPsych
Clinical Lecturer
Cardiff University

Psychotherapy
Dr Melanie F. Bowden MBBS, MRCPsych, MSc
Consultant Psychiatrist
Warneford Hospital, Oxford

Dr Anne-Marie Feeley MRCPsych
Specialist Registrar
Warneford Hospital, Oxford

Dr Karey Taylor BMBCh, MRCGP
Specialty Doctor
Warneford Hospital, Oxford

INTRODUCTION

THE CLINICAL ASSESSMENT OF SKILLS AND COMPETENCIES (CASC)

Since June 2008 the Royal College of Psychiatrists' membership examinations have taken the format of three written papers followed by a clinical examination, the Clinical Assessment of Skills and Competencies (CASC).

The CASC consists of 'stations'. A station is an encounter with an actor playing the role of a patient, relative or colleague. There is an examiner present. Sometimes there is another person in the booth who is an invigilator or a representative of a another Royal College. At the entrance to each station there is an information sheet pinned outside which contains some background on the simulated situation and instructions for the task. A candidate has to perform the task in a given time. This will usually involve taking a history, doing a risk assessment, performing an examination or giving information.

For examples of scenarios see the mock examination section at the back of this book. Timings are explained below.

Morning session: Four paired stations
    Two minutes preparation time
    Ten minutes doing the task
    Four paired stations = eight stations in total
    Total examination length = 1 hour 36 minutes

Afternoon session: Eight individual stations
    One minute preparation time
    Seven minutes doing the task
    Total examination length = 1 hour 4 minutes

In the morning because no one can start their circuit on the second station of a pair, there needs to be a staggered start. The first group of candidates go to the first station whilst the second group of candidates wait in silence until the one minute remaining bell sounds (after nine minutes). They then move silently to wait outside the first station. When the first group then moves onto their second station, the second group begin their first station. When the first group finish all of their stations, they will be asked to wait silently whilst the second group read the instructions for their last station. When the second group enter the booth of their last station, the first group will be led out of the examination hall in silence.

For both the morning and afternoon exams there may be pilot stations. These can be at any point during the examination, including at the start or the end, and will be in addition to the total examination time.

The examinations are likely to be run over several different days. As all of the examinations are identical on the same day, the candidates from each of the sessions need to be kept separate. This may mean that candidates can face a long wait before or after their examinations. Usually no electronic devices are allowed and you will be expected to hand in any you have brought. Written notes and books are usually permitted in the waiting period. Candidates are usually permitted to leave the examination venue at lunch time to return at a specified time for the afternoon session.

General tips
Before the examination
  Plan your journey well and consider traffic
  Think about staying in a hotel overnight
Take to the examination
  Any required ID
  Examination letter and/or entrance slip
  Adequate food and drink
  Study notes
For yourself
  Good personal hygiene
  Smart and conservative appearance
During the examination
  Smile appropriately
  Good introduction
    'Hello my name is 'Dr William Smith'
  Good explanation
    'I am one of the psychiatric doctors here and I would like to talk with you about what has
    been going on.'
  Gain permission
    'Are you happy to speak with me today?'
  Open and interested body language
  Use non-verbal communication such as nods and smiles
  Look interested
  Summarise back
  When giving information always ask what they already know
In all practical skills stations
  Make the patient comfortable
  Consider asking for a chaperone

HOW THE CASC IS MARKED

In each station the candidate will be assessed by a different examiner. This means that the
candidate's marks in any one station should not be affected by their performance in any other
station. If the candidate feels that they have performed badly in a station, they should remember
that each station is another opportunity to show a different examiner that they have the necessary
skills to pass the examination.

In each station the examiner is required to give a global rating of the candidate's performance.
Examiners give one of four grades:
  A (pass)
  B (borderline pass)
  C (borderline fail)
  D (fail).

Whilst there are four grades this is to aid the assessment of reliability of examiners. In essence
only a pass/fail decision is made.

Candidates are required to pass a certain number of stations in order to obtain an overall pass.

To help in assessing the global rating of the candidate, examiners are required to say if there were any areas of concern in the candidate's performance. For each station there are up to ten possible areas of concern. Examples of possible areas of concern include problems with:

1. Questioning style e.g. use of appropriate mix of open and closed questions
2. Listening and responding appropriately to interviewee/discussant
3. Management of interview/examination including empathic responses
4. Lack of appropriate focus for the required task
5. Fluency of interview/examination/discussion
6. Professionalism including but not limited to harmful interaction, failure to respect individual's rights, ethical behaviour etc.
7. Appropriate choice of avenues of enquiry, tests or examinations including significant omissions
8. Range and/or depth of history explored
9. Range and/or depth of psychopathology explored (signs elicited at examination)
10. Depth of enquiry into symptoms
11. Range and/or depth of risk explored
12. Appropriate application of cognitive testing
13. Analysis of problem and synthesis of opinion
14. Prioritisation, recognition of importance and appropriateness of information delivered and/or management.

The college has advised that areas of concern are marked for feedback reasons only and the number of areas of concern do not directly relate to the overall mark given.

KEY SKILLS

HOW TO USE THE KEY SKILLS SECTION

The key skills section contains four key skills as detailed below. Each of these skills may be relevant in any CASC station.

Differential diagnosis

Differential diagnosis is a key skill in the CASC. The differential diagnosis section shortens and simplifies the International Classification of Diseases (ICD-10) into an easier format, listing all the main categories and their major diagnoses. This information should enable candidates to see where different diagnoses fit together and to get used to the language of the ICD-10. Notable learning points include the use of the term 'hyperkinetic disorder', rather than 'ADHD', and the term 'emotionally unstable personality disorder, borderline type', rather than 'borderline personality disorder'.

Management

Being able to formulate sound management plans is a key skill in psychiatry; it is essential that the examiner feels that you are able to do this well. You may have a very good idea of what a management plan should include but, if your style is not up to scratch, you may come across as being under-confident and incompetent. This is why structure is so important. This section will help you develop an effective, pragmatic and logical management structure.

Risk

Demonstrating a safe working knowledge of risk assessment and management is an essential competency for the CASC examination. Candidates should consider risk issues in every CASC station just as they should consider risk in any clinical situation. This risk section includes approaches to the general assessment and management of risk as well as specific approaches to assessing and managing the risk of self harm, suicide, and violence. Whilst you will find that some stations in your CASC examination may prompt you to consider risk issues, there will be other instances where there may be no prompts. If there are no prompts, do not assume that you do not need to consider risk: you do not want to be seen as being an unsafe clinician just because you have misinterpreted the instructions. Likewise if the instructions clearly state that you do not need to perform a risk assessment do not waste your precious examination time in doing so: you will not score any extra marks but may annoy the examiner and lose marks for the actual task in hand. Where there is no mention of risk in the examination instructions, any risk assessment should of course be tailored to meet the needs of the task and should not take over all of your time in that station. You will notice that the individual topics in the *Topics* section of this book often do not make specific reference to risk; this is because the *Topics* section should be used *alongside* the key skills section.

Communication skills

Effective communications skills are absolutely crucial to the psychiatrist, and most people believe that the Royal College of Psychiatrists places an enormous emphasis on communication skills in their assessment of CASC examination candidates. Whilst communications skills are personal to the individual and may take many years to hone, this section will guide you through some common dos and don'ts and suggest ways to improve your interview skills.

COMMUNICATION SKILLS

You only have a few minutes to take a relevant history from the actor who is pretending to be a patient. It is vital to create good rapport quickly. Actors and patients may be more helpful if they like the candidate.

Appearance and manner

As in most psychiatric interviewing, the aim is to help the patient to feel comfortable. They will then usually do their best to be helpful. Greet the patient in a friendly way, for example: 'Hello, I am Dr William Smith.' Do not shake their hand unless the patient offers theirs. In some cultures hand shaking is not approved of, especially if a man shakes the hand of a woman. Remember to smile at appropriate times. This is easy to forget in a stressful situation, but it can make all the difference.

In the examination, dress conservatively. The majority of candidates wear a suit. Examination situations are not the time for extremes of dress or hair style.

Sit up straight to show alertness and interest in the patient. Do not cross your arms or legs for long periods as it appears defensive. Sitting with the knees held wide apart looks unprofessional. Do not lean so far forward that the patient feels uncomfortable.

Questioning style

In general, use mainly open questions early in the interview and closed questions to confirm points and to keep the patient on relevant subjects. Words such as 'what' and 'how' often start open questions, as well as 'Could you tell me more about that, please?' Sometimes it is very useful to repeat a significant word or phrase which the patient has used. For example you could say 'How else do the laser beams affect you?' or 'Could you tell me what you meant when you said you were "at the end of your tether"?' As with any interviewing technique, this should not be used so much that it annoys the other person.

Basic motivational interviewing techiques can be useful. For example, in a patient with an alcohol problem, consider a phrase such as 'what would have to happen for you to give up drinking?' This gives the patient the opportunity to mention their own solution, without the interviewer producing any new or jarring ideas. The patient's own ideas may be the best, as they know so much more of the background. Even if they are not the best, the patient is likely to value them more than the solutions produced by others.

It is best to speak in a simple way, without complicated medical expressions. This is particularly true when dealing with poorly-educated patients or those with learning disabilities. Echo the type of words they use. Such people have a much more limited vocabulary. The same is true when interviewing children, although you are unlikely to have to do this in the current examination.

The well-placed compliment

If the patient has succeeded at something, it can be useful, usually towards the end of an interview, to comment on it. An example of this would be 'I am impressed by how well you have kept your business going, with all that trouble at home'. Also, if the patient has done something useful to help solve their own problems, it is worth commenting on this too, so as remind them how they can help themselves more than they think and to improve their self esteem. For example, 'Your plan to return from work each day without passing the pub sounds a good one'. If the patient feels appreciated, they will value the interview more and may be better motivated to solve their own problems.

'That's right'

If the patient produces an important insight into their situation, it is very important for the interviewer to pay attention to it. One example might be: 'Taking street drugs has caused me so many problems that I really have to stop it for good'. A very useful comment from the interviewer would be 'That's right.' This reply confirms the patient's point of view in an inconspicuous but very significant way. It uses simple vocabulary familiar even to young children and therefore it may enter the patient's understanding at a deep level.

Mirroring

People who are getting on well when talking together often adopt a similar posture and manner. Their tones of voice may also mirror each other, for example they both speak quickly or slowly, loudly or softly, and they are both either happy or sad. They do this quite naturally, without thinking about it. The skilled interviewer can use this technique deliberately to improve rapport by making the patient feel more relaxed and accepted. The technique must not be done in an obvious way, as this can be threatening for the patient.

Dealing with anger

Modelling can be used to lead someone to a more satisfactory state of mind. If the patient is angry, for example, the interviewer can model a less aroused manner.

When someone is angry, there is often at least some justification for their feelings. If you show that you appreciate this, it helps to lessen their aggression. Only say you agree with those points with which you think are true. The more you agree with the patient, the less they have to be angry about.

Conversation during the examination

The examination is usually held in a large hall with a high ceiling, such as a sports centre. There will be more than a hundred other people in the room. Naturally there is quite a bit of background noise.

A depressed person may speak rather quietly, so you may wish to speak a little quieter than usual. However remember to speak loudly enough to be heard by both the actor-patient and the examiner. It is not good to shout, as this may intimidate the patient and even disturb the people in the neighbouring booth.

Answer the question

You have one minute in the individual stations and two minutes in the linked stations to read the instructions pinned outside the booth. It is most important to follow what they say. When you are in the booth, if you want to check what the sheet said, there is a copy in the booth and the examiner will show you where it is. If the instructions say 'Do a risk assessment', then do just that, and remember that there may be several people who could be vulnerable, not just one.

Marking

Each station is marked individually and some are harder than others. If you think you have not done well in one booth, put it behind you and concentrate on the next question. Even if you have not passed every station, you may still pass the examination.

REFERENCES

Poole, R. & Higgo, R. (2006) *Psychiatric Interviewing and Assessment*. Cambridge University Press.

Organic disorders (F00–F09)
- F00   Dementia in Alzheimer's disease
- F01   Vascular dementia
- F02   Dementia in other diseases
- F04   Organic amnesic syndrome
- F07   Personality and behavioural disorder due to brain disease, damage or dysfunction

Disorders due to psychoactive substance use (F10–F19)
Each group of psychoactive substances has its own prefix (e.g. F10.x = alcohol). All groups share following prefixes
- F1x.0   Acute intoxication
- F1x.1   Harmful use
- F1x.2   Dependence syndrome
- F1x.3   Withdrawal state
- F1x.4   Withdrawal state with delirium
- F1x.5   Psychotic disorder
- F1x.6   Amnesic syndrome

Schizophrenia, schizotypal and delusional disorders (F20–F29)
- F20   Schizophrenia
  - F20.0   Paranoid
  - F20.1   Hebephrenic
- F21   Schizotypal disorder
- F22   Persistent delusional disorders
- F23   Acute and transient psychotic disorders
- F24   Induced delusional disorder
- F25   Schizoaffective disorders

Mood (affective) disorders (F30–F39)
- F30   Manic episode
  - F30.0   Hypomania
  - F30.1   Mania without psychotic symptoms
  - F30.2   Mania with psychotic symptoms
- F31   Bipolar affective disorder
- F32   Depressive episode
- F33   Recurrent depressive disorder
- F34   Persistent mood (affective) disorder
  - F34.0   Cyclothymia
  - F34.1   Dysthymia

Neurotic, stress-related and somatoform disorders (F40–F49)
- F40   Phobic anxiety disorders
  - F40.0   Agoraphobia
  - F40.1   Social phobias
- F41   Other anxiety disorders
  - F41.0   Panic disorder
  - F41.1   Generalised anxiety disorder
- F42   Obsessive—compulsive disorder
- F43   Reaction to severe stress, and adjustment disorders
  - F43.0   Acute stress reaction
  - F43.1   Post-traumatic stress disorder
  - F43.2   Adjustment disorders

F44   Dissociative [conversion] disorders

F45   Somatoform disorders

Behavioural syndromes associated with physical factors (F50–F59)

F50   Eating disorders

    F50.0   Anorexia nervosa

    F50.2   Bulimia nervosa

F51   Non-organic sleep disorders

F52   Non-organic sexual dysfunction

F53   Mental and behavioural disorders associated with the puerperium

Disorders of adult personality and behaviour (F60–F69)

F60   Specific personality disorders

    F60.0   Paranoid personality disorder

    F60.1   Schizoid personality disorder

    F60.2   Dissocial personality disorder

    F60.3   Emotionally unstable personality disorder

        F60.30   Impulsive type

        F60.31   Borderline type

F62   Enduring personality changes

F63   Habit and impulse disorders

    F63.0   Pathological gambling

F64   Gender identity disorders

F65   Disorders of sexual preference

    F65.0   Fetishism

    F65.2   Exhibitionism

    F65.4   Paedophilia

F68   Other disorders of adult personality and behaviour

    F68.1   Factitious disorder

Mental retardation (F70–F79)

F70   Mild mental retardation (50–69)

F71   Moderate mental retardation (35–49)

F72   Severe mental retardation (20–34)

F73   Profound mental retardation (<20)

Disorders of psychological development (F80–F89)

F80   Specific development disorders of speech and language

F81   Specific development disorders of scholastic skills

F84   Pervasive developmental disorders

    F84.0   Childhood autism

    F84.5   Asperger's syndrome

Behavioural and emotional disorders with onset usually occurring in childhood and adolescence (F90–F99)

F90   Hyperkinetic disorder

F91   Conduct disorders

    F91.3   Oppositional defiant disorder

F93   Emotional disorders with onset specific to childhood

F94   Disorders of social functioning with onset specific to childhood and adolescence

F95   Tic disorders

REFERENCES

Cooper, J. (ed.) (2004) *Pocket Guide to the ICD-10: Classification of Mental and Behavioural Disorders*. Churchill Livingstone.

MANAGEMENT

Information gathering
Sources of information
    Patient
    Collateral history
    GP records
    Hospital records
    Inmate medical records (IMR)
    School

Delivery
Location
    Home
    GP surgery
    Day hospital
    Open psychiatric wards (general, rehabilitation)
    Closed psychiatric wards [Psychiatric Intensive Care Units (PICU), seclusion]
    Secure units (low, medium or high)
    Medical ward
Input
    Primary care
    Outpatient clinic
    Community Mental Health Team (CMHT)
    Crisis Resolution Home Treatment Team
    Assertive Outreach Team
    Rehabilitation Team
    Early Intervention in Psychosis Team (EIP)
CPA
    4 key components
        Assessment
        Care plan
        Care coordinator
        Regular review

Psychological
Immediate
    Anxiety management techniques
    Counselling services
    Telephone helplines (e.g. Samaritans)
    Drop in centres (e.g. AA)
    Self-help books (Bibliotherapy)
    Behavioural techniques (Antecedent → Behaviour → Consequences)
Long term
    Cognitive Behavioural Therapy (CBT)
    Cognitive Analytic Therapy (CAT)
    Dialectical Behavioural Therapy (DBT)
    Individual Psychodynamic Psychotherapy
    Brief Solution Focused Psychotherapy
    Psychoanalysis
    Family therapy

Biological
Immediate
   Medication
      Hypnotics, anxiolytics, rapid tranquilisation
   Physical investigations
      Observations (pulse, BP, temp, weight)
      Examination (CVR, GI, CNS, thyroid)
      Bloods (glucose, U&Es, LFTs, TFTs, Ca, FBC, Cu, B_{12}, folate, Mg)
      Neuroimaging (CT, MRI)
      Urine dipstick
      Drug screen
   Physical treatments
      Of underlying physical problems
      Emergency ECT, re-feeding
Long term
   Medication
      Psychotropic (oral vs. depot)
      Treatment of side effects
   Physical investigations
      CSF, SPECT, EEG, Bone Density Scan,
      Penile Plesmography (PPG)
   Monitoring
      Bloods (LFTs, TFTs, U&Es, FBC, prolactin,
      drug plasma levels, glucose, lipids)
      ECG, BMI
   Physical treatments
      Of underlying physical problems
      ECT, psychosurgery (rare)

Social
Immediate
   Simple advice (sleep hygiene)
   Psychoeducation
   Childcare
   Emergency accommodation
   Driving (DVLA advice)
Long term
   Voluntary sector (MIND, drug support)
   Support groups (including carer support)
   Accommodation (independent vs. supported)
   Benefits [Disability Living Allowance (DLA), Incapacity Benefit]
   Working to meeting cultural needs

RISK

Key terms
Static risk factors
   Factors which are unlikely to change e.g. past criminal history.
Dynamic risk factors
   Factors which can change over time e.g. substance misuse.
Actuarial risk assessment
   Risk assessment based upon statistical calculations of probability. Usually carried out using actuarial risk assessment tools.
Clinical risk assessment
   Risk assessment based on clinical appraisal of factors related to risk. Sometimes carried out using clinical risk assessment guides.

Risk factors
Previous history
   This may be the most important
Personal factors
   Demographics e.g. gender, age, marital status
   Personality
   Employment status
Illness related factors
   Psychosis
   Substance misuse
   Treatment resistance
   Compliance
Present mental state
   Appearance/behaviour, speech, mood, thoughts, perceptions, insight, cognition
Situational factors
   Type of employment
   Proximity to vulnerable people (children, LD, elderly)

Risk posed
To self
   Deliberate self harm, suicide, neglect
   Sexual, physical, emotional, financial
To or from other adults
   Sexual, physical, emotional, financial exploitation
Children/vulnerable Adults
   Sexual, physical, emotional, financial exploitation, neglect
Property
   Private vs. public
   Fire-setting, neglect, security, safety

Risk assessment tools
Violence
   HCR-20 (Historical Clinical Risk-20)
   VRAG (Violence Risk and Appraisal Guide)
Sexual Offending
   SVR-20 (Sexual Violent Risk-20)
Spousal Risk
   SARA (Spousal Assault Risk Assessment Guide)
Suicide
   Beck Suicide Intent Scale

Principles of risk management
Multi agency involvement
    Service user/carer
    Multidisciplinary team (MDT)
    Police
    Probation
    Multi-Agency Public Protection Arrangements (MAPPA)
Information sharing
    Risk registers
        Vulnerable adult, sex offender, child protection

ASSESSING RISK OF DELIBERATE SELF HARM AND SUICIDE

Risk factors
Previous history
    History of previous deliberate self harm/suicide attempts
    Previous psychiatric history
Personal factors
    Old age
    Unemployment
    Single, widowed, or separated
    Lack of supportive social network
Psychiatric and medical factors
    Personality disorder
    Substance misuse
    Mood disorder
    Schizophrenia
    Chronic painful illness
Factors in the mental state
    Low mood
    Marked hopelessness
    Thoughts of self harm
    Plans to harm self
    Hallucinations commanding harm to self

Assessing current situation
Low mood and marked hopelessness
    'What is your mood like?'
    'What do you think will happen to you in the future?'
Thoughts of self harm
    'I am sorry to hear you have not been feeling very well.'
    'Sometimes, when people become low in mood, thoughts of self harm can creep in. Has this
    happened to you?'
    'Sometimes people feel that they would be better off if they weren't here anymore. Have you
    ever felt like that?'
    'Has anything happened recently to make you feel this way?'
Plans to harm self
    'Have ever thought about acting on these thoughts?'
    'Have you made any specific plans?'
    'What do they involve?'
Hallucinations commanding harm to self
    'Sometimes people hear voices when there is no one else around. Has this ever happened to
    you?'
        'Have these voices ever given you any instructions?'
        'Tell me about these instructions.'
        'Why do you feel that you must follow these instructions?'
Substance misuse
    'How much alcohol do you drink?'
    'Have you ever taken any illegal drugs?'
    'Could you tell me a bit about this?'

Assessing previous suicide attempt
Previous history
    'Have you ever harmed yourself or tried to take your own life?'

Beck Suicide Intent Scale
  Isolation
    'Where did you take the overdose?'
    'Was anyone present when you took the overdose?'
    'Were they in the same room?'
  Timing
    'Did you expect to be found in time?'
  Precautions against discovery and/or intervention
    'Did you barricade yourself in or lock the door?'
  Acting to gain help during or after the attempt
    'Did you inform anyone of what you had done after the attempt?'
  Final acts in anticipation of death
    'Did you leave any gifts or write a will?'
  Degree of planning for suicide attempt
    'Did you prepare and make plans for the overdose?'
  Suicide note
    'Did you leave a note?'
  Overt communication of intent before act
    'Did you tell anyone about the overdose before taking it?'
  Purpose of attempt
    'Why did you take the overdose?' (to manipulate the environment, for attention, for revenge, to solve problems)
  Expectations regarding fatality of act
    'Did you expect to die?'
  Conception of method's fatality
    'Did you think that the overdose would kill you?'
    'Did you think it would harm you?'
  Seriousness of attempt
    'How serious were you about the attempt?'
  Ambivalence towards living
    'How do you feel about the attempt now?'
  Concept of medical reversibility
    'Did you think that the doctors and nurses would be able to save you?'
  Degree of premeditation
    'Did you do it on the spur of the moment or did you plan it?'

Essential guidelines (NICE guidelines 2004)

All people who self harm should be offered a full mental health assessment and a thorough risk assessment.

REFERENCES
Beck, A.T. et al. (1974). *The Prediction of Suicide*. Charles Press, Philadelphia.
NICE Clinical Guidelines (2004). *The Short-Term Physical and Psychological Management and Secondary Prevention of Self-Harm in Primary and Secondary Care*. National Institute for Clinical Excellence.

ASSESSING RISK OF VIOLENCE

Risk factors
Previous history
  History of previous violence
  History of impulsive behaviour
Personal factors
  Male and young
  Unemployment
  Divorced or separated
  Lack of supportive social network
Psychiatric and medical factors
  Personality disorder
  Psychopathy
  Substance misuse
  Psychotic symptoms
Factors in mental state
  Thoughts of harming others
  Plans to harm others
  Delusions of persecution, jealousy or control
  Hallucinations commanding harm to others
Situational factors
  Availability of weapon
  Access to potential victim
  Difficult relationship with potential victim

Assessing current situation
Thoughts of harming others
  'Have you ever had thoughts about harming someone else?'
  'Tell me about those thoughts.'
Plans to harm others
  'Have ever thought about acting on these thoughts?'
  'Have you made any specific plans?'
  'What do they involve?'
Delusions of persecution, control or jealousy
  'Has anything strange been happening recently?'
  'Sometimes people who have thoughts of harming others are afraid of something, such as feeling that someone wants to do them harm. Have you ever felt like that?'
  'Have you ever felt as if you are being controlled by someone else?'
    'Have you ever felt as if someone else is in control of your thoughts?'
  'Are you in a relationship?'
    'Are there any problems with your relationship which is making you feel this way?'
Hallucinations commanding harm to others
  'Sometimes people hear voices when there is no one else around. Has this ever happened to you?'
    'Have these voices ever given you any instructions?'
    'Tell me about these instructions.'
    'Why do you feel that you must follow these instructions?'
Substance misuse
  'How much alcohol do you drink?'
  'Have you ever taken any illegal drugs?'
  'Could you tell me a bit about this?'

Assessing previous violence

Previous history
   'Have you ever harmed anyone?'
What
   'What happened?'
Who
   'Who did you hurt?'
How
   'Did you attack him with your fists or did you use a weapon?'
Where
   'Where did this happen?'
When
   'How old were you at the time?'
Why
   'Why did you hurt him?'
   'Was the attack provoked or was it out of the blue?'
   'Was there anything going on in your life at this time?'
   'Were you drunk at the time of the violence?'
      'Had you been taking drugs?'
   'Sometimes people who are violent describe hearing voices telling them to harm others. Were you hearing similar things around this time?'
      'What did the voices say?'
      'Why did you have to do what they said?'
   'Sometimes people who harm others do so because they believe that they are under threat. Did you feel threatened at this time?'
      'Can you tell me how you felt threatened?'
      'Did you tell anyone about it?'
      'What do you think would have happened if you had told someone about it?'
Planning
   'Did you plan to hurt him or did it happen out of the blue?'
Remorse
   'Do you think he deserved it?'
   'Did you regret hurting him?'
Other previous history
   'Have you ever hurt anyone else?'
      'Could you tell me more about this?'
   'How old were you when you first became violent?'
Forensic history
   'Has your violence ever got you into trouble with the law?'
   'Have you ever been charged or convicted of a violent offence?'
History of impulsive behaviour
   'Have you ever taken unnecessary chances or done reckless things?'
      'When you took these chances did you think about the consequences?'

Essential guidelines (NICE guidelines 2005)

The assessment of a service user's risk of violence should be ongoing and should include the views of the service user and if possible, his carer.

REFERENCES

Gelder, M., Harrison, P. & Cowen, P. (2001) *Shorter Oxford Textbook of Psychiatry*. Fifth Edn. Oxford University Press. pp. 52–53 & 314–316.

NICE Clinical Guidelines (2005). *The Short-Term Management of Disturbed/Violent Behaviour in Psychiatric In-patient Settings and Emergency Departments*. National Institute for Clinical Excellence.

TOPICS

HOW TO USE THE TOPICS SECTION

The CASC is about more than demonstrating clinical knowledge. The Royal College is clear in its view that candidates who approach CASC stations with a checklist method are unlikely to do well, which implies that it expects a rounded demonstration of clinical skills and competencies. Whilst you cannot afford to let yourself concentrate solely on demonstrating your clinical knowledge in each CASC station, you equally cannot afford to be ill-prepared.

This topics section is designed to give you a user-friendly overview of the examinable areas of psychiatry as laid out in the current MRCPsych CASC Blueprint. These areas are general adult, old age, child and adolescent, learning disability, psychotherapy and forensic. Our topic section covers these six areas and also includes a section on substance misuse. Other potential areas such as liaison psychiatry are covered too, but rather than being given a specific section of their own, the relevant information is found in other areas such as general adult or practical skills. In addition to these seven clinical subspecialties, the topics section also includes a section entitled 'Practical skills', where guidance on physical examinations and investigations may be found, and a section entitled 'Legislation and resources', where you will find information on the Mental Health Act, capacity and mental health resources. The information contained in each topic is geared to the sort of information that you will expect to encounter in any given CASC station. It is important to note that this section is not a substitute for a textbook and you will find that you may want to refer to a textbook as part of your examination preparation.

You will find that some topics are presented differently to others. This is because it is recognised that certain topics are examined differently to others. For example, whereas some topics may suggest ways of explaining management to patients, others will be more focussed towards the discussion of management with colleagues. However, at the same time you will notice that there are themes which run throughout the topics section, some of these are detailed below.

Core diagnostic criteria

You are expected to demonstrate a sound working knowledge of diagnostic criteria. Wherever you see the subheading core diagnostic criteria, you will find the core criteria from the ICD-10. Learning all the ICD-10 criteria for every possible diagnosis is, of course, unrealistic. It is far more important to understand the main criteria for key diagnoses and how these fit together.

Key phrases

Candidates often find it difficult to know how to phrase questions and how to put psychiatric terms into everyday language. As clear and empathetic communication is so important in the CASC, you will find that many of the topics in this section include key phrases which are identified with quotation marks. Whilst it is not expected that candidates should learn these key phrases off by heart, we do hope that they will offer a useful starting point. You may even find that you can adapt certain phrases to suit a range of different scenarios.

Information giving

Information giving is a difficult skill to master for the purposes of the CASC. Because time is so limited, it is very easy to panic and feel that you must tell the patient as much as you can as quickly as you can. This approach will lose you marks as it will look as if you are just regurgitating a set of lecture notes. Information giving is a two-way process and a skilled clinician will ask the patient what they already know and will ask the patient to stop them at any time. It can also be useful to ask the patient to summarise what you have told them so that you can be sure that they understand what may be a very difficult concept or management plan. Sometimes you will see that the Information-giving section is aimed at fellow professionals and not at the patient, this is usually because it is expected that the topic is more likely to be examined in a CASC station where the actor is playing a fellow professional than a patient or relative.

Essential guidelines

Evidence-based medicine is a key principle in modern medicine. Therefore it is important that you can demonstrate a working knowledge of the Essential guidelines such as the NICE guidelines in your management of mental illness. However, it is also recognised that examination preparation time is often limited. With this in mind, this section has been written to help familiarise you with some of these most recent essential guidelines.

Some topics, such as forensic mental health legislation, lend themselves better to an information sheet structure. Whilst it is most unlikely that you will ever encounter a CASC station dedicated to a topic such as forensic mental health legislation, a topic such as this may nonetheless be examined as part of another topic such as pathological jealousy.

It is important also to note that references to the third person are always masculine i.e. he, him and his, except in instances where this would be inappropriate, e.g. in relation to pregnancy or breastfeeding. This is to prevent the clumsy use of terms such as 's/he', which may prove distracting for some readers. For similar reasons, you will find the term 'patient' favoured throughout this book. There is much debate on this subject and more recently the term 'service-user' has become common place. Essentially the choice is yours.

PSYCHOSIS

Key phrases

Disorder of the content of thought (delusions)
    Persecutory
        'Is anyone trying to harm you?'
        'Is anyone spying on you?'
        'Are there any plots or conspiracies that you know about?'
    Reference
        'Do you see any reference to yourself on TV?'
        'Are things ever arranged to have a special meaning?'
    Guilt
        'Do you feel you have done anything wrong?'
    Grandiosity
        'Do you have any special talents, powers or abilities?'
    Nihilism
        'Do you feel something terrible has happened or will?'
    Hypochondriasis
        'How's your health?'
    Delusional mood
        'Is there anything strange going on that concerns you?'
    Delusional misidentification
        'Are there people about who are not what they seem or who are in disguise?'
    Delusion of love
        'Are you loved by anyone who does not publicly acknowledge it?'
    Delusions of passivity
        'Is there any kind of outside control over your feelings, impulses or actions?'
        'Do you ever feel like a zombie, a robot, or a puppet?'
        Passivity of emotion (made to feel)
        'Is there anything or anyone making you feel a certain way?'
        Passivity of thought (made to think)
        'Is there anything or anyone making you think a certain way?'
        Passivity of action (made to do)
        'Do you feel that your will has been replaced by that of some outside force?'
        Somatic passivity
        'Do you think that someone or something produces strange experiences of your body?'
Disorder of the form of thought (formal thought disorder)
    Evident from speech
        'Are you able to think clearly?'
Disorder of the possession of thought
    Thought insertion
        'Do you have any thoughts which are not your own?'
    Thought withdrawal
        'Are you thoughts ever taken from your mind?'
        'Do your thoughts sometimes suddenly stop?'
    Thought broadcasting
        'Do your thoughts become public somehow?'
        'Can people access your thoughts?'
        'Do your thoughts seem aloud in your head?'

Disorder of perception (hallucinations)
'Have you had any odd or unpleasant experiences lately?'
Auditory hallucinations
'Do you ever hear noises or voices when there is nobody about and no ordinary explanation?'
Establishing whether second or third person: 'Does the voice speak to you or about you?'
Running commentary: 'Some people experience voices which describe what they are doing. Have you had a similar experience?'
Thought echo: 'Do you ever hear your thoughts spoken aloud?'
Visual hallucinations
'Have you ever had visions or seen things other people couldn't?'
Gustatory hallucinations
'Have you noticed any unusual or unpleasant tastes?'
Olfactory hallucinations
'Have you noticed any unusual smells?'
Tactile hallucinations
'Do you have any unusual sexual sensations?'
'Do you notice any strange sensations of touch, temperature, pain?'
'Have you experienced any crawling sensation under the skin?'
Special kinds of hallucinations to consider
Functional
Reflex
Extracampine
Autoscopy or phantom mirror-image
Hypnagogic and hypnopompic
Insight
'What do you think about these experiences?

Some organic causes of psychosis
Drug-induced
Electrolyte disturbances
Hyponatraemia
Hypomagnesaemia
Hypocalcaemia
Hypercalcaemia
Hypoglycaemia
Sepsis
Hepatic encephalopathy
Delirium
Dementia
AIDS
Brain tumours

REFERENCES

Gelder, M., Harrison, P. & Cowen, P. (2001) *Shorter Oxford Textbook of Psychiatry*. (5th edn) Oxford University Press p27
Casey, P. & Kelly, B. (2007) *Fish's Clinical Psychopathology: Signs and Symptoms in Psychiatry* (3rd edn) Gaskell
Poole, R. & Higgo, R. (2006) *Psychiatric Interviewing and Assessment* Cambridge University Press
Sims, A. *Symptoms in the Mind: an Introduction to Descriptive Psychopathology* (2nd edn) W.B. Saunders

SCHIZOPHRENIA AND SCHIZOTYPAL DISORDER

Core diagnostic criteria (ICD-10)

Schizophrenia
  General criteria (1 month of symptoms)
  1 of
    Thought insertion/withdrawal/broadcasting/echo
    Delusions of control/influence/passivity/delusional perceptions
  or 2 of
    Persistent hallucinations in any modality (accompanied by delusions or by persistent overvalued ideas)
    Neologisms/loss of train of thought resulting in incoherent speech
    Catatonic behaviour (posturing; waxy flexibility; negativism; mutism; stupor)
    Negative symptoms (marked apathy; paucity of speech; blunting of affect)
  Paranoid schizophrenia
    Dominated by relatively stable, often paranoid delusions which are usually accompanied by hallucinations and perceptual disturbances
  Hebephrenic schizophrenia
    Dominated by shallow and inappropriate affect, disorganised thought and incoherent speech
  Catatonic schizophrenia
    Dominated by prominent and sustained catatonic behaviour
  Residual schizophrenia
    A late stage of schisophrenia characterised by long-term negative symptoms
  Simple schizophrenia
    Characterised by an insidious development of oddities of conduct, inability to meet demands of society and decline in total performance without prior psychotic symptoms
Schizotypal disorder
  A disorder in which the eccentric behaviour and anomalies of thinking and affect resemble schizophrenia, but which do not meet the diagnostic criteria. Clinical features:
    Inappropriate affect, which makes individual appear cold
    Odd, eccentric or peculiar behaviour
    Poor rapport with others and tendency to social withdrawal
    Odd beliefs or magical thinking
    Suspiciousness or paranoid ideas
    Ruminations without inner resistance
    Unusual perceptual experiences (e.g. somatosensory illusions)
    Vague, circumstantial thinking and odd speech
    Occasional quasipsychotic episodes

Information giving

What is schizophrenia?
  'Schizophrenia is a treatable mental illness. It affects thinking, emotions and behaviour.'
  'It affects 1 person in every 100 during their lifetime. People usually develop schizophrenia between the ages of 15 and 35. The symptoms can be controlled with treatment: however, it can often last a long time and can be very disabling.'
What causes it?
  'No-one knows for sure. There seem to be a number of different causes.'
  'Schizophrenia tends to run in families. Genes provide about half of the explanation. Some affected people have changes in the structure of their brains. Some may have had viral infections or problems during birth.'

'Using illicit drugs can bring on schizophrenia in someone who is already at risk of developing the illness.'

'Growing up in inner cities seems to increase the chances of developing it.'

'In people with schizophrenia certain chemical messengers in the brain, called neurotransmitters do not work correctly. One of these neurotransmitters is called dopamine.'

'Although stressful events may not cause schizophrenia they can bring on the illness. Long term stress such as family tension may also make it worse.'

Is it a split mind?

'No. Some people believe that someone with schizophrenia can be normal one minute and turn violent the next. This is not true. People with schizophrenia are rarely dangerous. People with schizophrenia can have trouble distinguishing between what is real and what is not.'

Medication

'The medications for schizophrenia are called antipsychotics. They help to reduce symptoms by correcting a chemical imbalance in the brain.'

'Older antipsychotic drugs called "typicals" can cause side effects such as stiffness and restlessness. These are usually reversible. However people sometimes get permanent abnormal movements of the mouth and tongue. This is called tardive dyskinesia and it affects 1 in 20 people.'

'Newer antipsychotic drugs called "atypicals" can cause sexual problems, weight gain, and possibly diabetes.'

'They all work by regulating the chemical messengers in the brain. Medication should be continued indefinitely in most people to prevent symptoms coming back. Some people find it easier to take the medication in injection form once every two, three or four weeks.'

What support is available?

'There is lots of support available, whether in hospital or in the community. We work as a team. There are psychiatrists, nurses, social workers, psychologists, occupational therapists and support workers who are available to work with you.'

'These professionals work together to support patients as well as their families. They each have different areas of expertise to help make your life as good as possible.'

Driving

'The DVLA says that people who have schizophrenia must be well and stable for at least three months before they may be allowed to drive again. This means that you must take medications regularly and must not be suffering from any side-effects which would make driving unsafe.'

Essential guidelines (NICE guidelines on schizophrenia 2002)

Use atypical antipsychotics as first line treatment at the lower end of BNF dose range.

If using typical antipsychotics, use 300–1000mg chlorpromazine dose equivalent.

Depot antipsychotics should be considered where there is covert non-compliance with an oral antipsychotic drug.

Clozapine should be considered if there is no significant improvement after at least two antipsychotics (including one atypical) have each been used for six to eight weeks.

REFERENCES

Cooper, J. (ed.) (2004) *Pocket Guide to the ICD-10: Classification of Mental and Behavioural Disorders.* Churchill Livingstone pp. 92–105

Gelder, M., Harrison, P. & Cowen, P. (2001) *Shorter Oxford Textbook of Psychiatry* (5th edn) Oxford University Press pp. 267–306

Johnstone, E.C. & Cunningham Owens, D.G. et al. (eds) (2004) *Companion to Psychiatric Studies* (7th edn) Churchill Livingstone pp. 390–420.

NICE Clinical Guidelines: Schizophrenia core interventions in the treatment and management of schizophrenia in primary and secondary care. National Institute for Clinical Excellence (2002)

BIPOLAR AFFECTIVE DISORDER

For depression aspect, see next section, *Depression and persistent mood (affective) disorders.*

Core diagnostic criteria (ICD-10)

Hypomania
  Mood is mildly elevated
  Symptoms do not lead to severe disruption or work or social rejection
Mania
  Mood is elevated out of keeping with the patient's circumstances
  Symptoms may result in behaviour that is inappropriate and reckless
Mania with psychotic symptoms
  In addition to mania there are delusions (usually grandiose) or hallucinations (usually second person)
Symptoms
  Increased activity or physical restlessness
  Increased talkativeness (pressure of speech in mania)
  Difficulty in concentration or distractibility (flight of ideas in mania)
  Decreased need for sleep
  Increased sexual energy
  Overspending or other reckless behaviour (pronounced in mania)
  Increased sociability or over familiarity
  Increased self-esteem or grandiosity
Mixed affective state
  Mixture or rapid alternation (within few hours) of hypomanic, manic and depressive symptoms

Key phrases

Mood
  'How would you describe your mood?'
  'How long has it been like that?'
  'Have you felt more irritable lately?'
  'Have you had more arguments than usual?'
Increased activity or physical restlessness
  'How is your energy?'
  'Do you feel full of energy?'
Increased talkativeness (pressure of speech in mania)
  Observe speech for pressure of speech
Difficulty in concentration or distractibility (flight of ideas in mania)
  'How is your concentration?'
  'Are you easily distracted?'
  'Do your thoughts ever seem to race?'
Decreased need for sleep
  'How is your sleep?'
  'How much sleep do you need?'
  'Have you been sleeping more than usual or less than usual?'
Increased sexual energy
  'How is your sex drive?'
  'Has it always been the same?'
  'Have you had any recent sexual encounters?'
Overspending or other reckless behaviour (pronounced in mania)

'Have you been spending more than usual?'
'Have you made any luxury purchases?'
'Have you spent more than you can afford?'
'When were you last at work?'
'Have you missed anytime off work?'
'Have you felt full of exciting ideas?'
Increased sociability or over familiarity
'Do you feel more friendly than usual?'
'Have you been socialising more than usual?'
Increased self-esteem or grandiosity
'How do you feel about yourself?'
'Do you feel confident?'
'Do you have any special powers or amazing talents?'

Information giving

Description
'We all experience minor changes in our mood from one day to the next or from one week to the next. Generally, our mood is an appropriate response to the events in our lives at the time.'
'People who have bipolar affective disorder tend to have major changes in mood for no obvious reason. They may be extremely excited or happy when there is no reason to be.'
'At the other extreme is depression, where low mood, reduced levels of energy and loss of interest may be experienced.'
'In bipolar affective disorder, the mood can switch between these two mood states.'
'It can be very disruptive to the affected person's life and those around them.'
'Sometimes, people with bipolar affective disorder will think in a disordered way and may hold strange and false beliefs.'
Prognosis
'Both the episodes and the length of time for which people remain well between episodes vary from one person to the next.'
'The pattern of the changes from one mood state to another also varies between people. For example older people have an increased risk of depression after mania.'
'Some people might have two to three episodes during a lifetime, while others will have four or more episodes a year.'
'Fortunately, with regular medication, we can reduce or even prevent further episodes of the illness.'
Epidemiology
'About 1 in 100 people will develop this illness at some time in their lives, usually starting before the age of 30, although the illness can start after this age.'
Treatment
Mood stabilizers
Antipsychotics
Support groups
The Manic Depression Fellowship

Essential guidelines (NICE guidelines on bipolar disorder 2006)

Short term management
If not on any medication
Use an antipsychotic
If no response add in lithium or valproate

If on medication
  Check dose and/or plasma levels
  Consider adding in an antipsychotic if levels of medication in range
Long term management
  Step one
    Lithium or valproate or olanzapine
  Step two
    Combination of the drugs in step one
  Step three
    Lamotrigine or carbamazepine

REFERENCES

Cooper, J. (ed) (2004) *Pocket Guide to the ICD-10: Classification of Mental and Behavioural Disorders.* Churchill Livingstone pp. 125–131

Gelder, M., Harrison, P. & Cowen, P. (2001) *Shorter Oxford Textbook of Psychiatry* (5th edn) Oxford University Press pp. 217–265

Johnstone, EC. & Cunningham Owens, DG. et al. (eds) *Companion to Psychiatric Studies* (7th edn) Churchill Livingstone pp. 421–449

NICE Clinical Guidelines: Bipolar disorder the management of bipolar disorder in adults, children and adolescents, in primary and secondary care. National Institute for Clinical Excellence (2006)

DEPRESSION AND PERSISTENT MOOD (AFFECTIVE) DISORDERS

Core diagnostic criteria (ICD-10)

Mild depressive episode
> Two or three symptoms are usually present. The patient is usually distressed by these but will probably be able to continue with most activities.

Moderate depressive episode
> Four or more symptoms are usually present. The patient is likely to have great difficulty in continuing with ordinary activities.

Severe depressive episode without psychotic symptoms
> Several of the symptoms are present and they are marked and distressing. Loss of self-esteem, ideas of worthlessness or guilt, suicidal ideas or acts are common, and symptoms of the somatic syndrome are usually present.

Severe depressive episode without psychotic symptoms
> As above but with the presence of hallucinations, delusions, psychomotor retardation or stupor so severe that ordinary social activities are impossible. The hallucinations or delusions may or may not be mood-congruent.

Symptoms
> Low mood
> Decreased interests or pleasures
> Decreased energy or fatigue
> Disturbed sleep
> Decreased appetite or weight loss
> Psychomotor retardation or agitation
> Decreased confidence or self esteem
> Guilt or self reproach
> Decreased concentration
> Deliberate self harm or suicidal ideation

Symptoms of the somatic syndrome
> Mood worse in the morning
> Decreased interests or pleasures
> Early morning wakening
> Decreased appetite or weight loss
> Psychomotor retardation or agitation
> Decreased emotional reactivity
> Decreased libido

Cyclothymia
> Persistent instability of mood involving numerous periods of depression and mild elation, but does not meet the diagnostic criteria for bipolar affective disorder or depression

Dysthymia
> Chronic depression of mood which lasts at least several years but which is not severe or prolonged enough to meet the diagnostic criteria for depression

Key phrases

Low mood
> 'How would you describe your mood?'
> 'How long have you been feeling this way?'
> 'Do you feel like this all day?'
> 'Do you feel worse at certain times of the day?'

Decreased interests or pleasures
  'What do you enjoy doing?'
  'Did you used to do other things?'
Decreased energy or fatigue
  'How are your energy levels?'
  'Do you have the same 'get up and go' that you used to?'
Disturbed sleep
  'How is your sleep?'
  'Do you have trouble getting off to sleep?'
  'Do you ever wake in the night or early in the morning?'
Decreased appetite or weight loss
  'How is your appetite?'
  'Has your weight changed?'
Decreased confidence or self-esteem
  'How do you feel about yourself?'
  'How is your confidence?'
Guilt or self reproach
  'Have you ever felt guilty?'
Decreased concentration
  'Are you able to concentrate?'
  'Can you follow the plot in a film or book?'
Deliberate self-harm or suicidal ideation
  'Have you ever thought about harming yourself?'
  'Have things ever got that bad that you have felt like ending it all?'
  'Have you made any plans?'
Decreased libido
  'May I ask you a personal question?'
  'Has your sex drive been affected?'
Decreased emotional reactivity
  'Some people who feel depressed sometimes find that they feel less love for their close ones, have you felt like that?'
Screen for psychotic type
  Delusions: Guilt
      'Do you feel you have done anything wrong?'
  Delusions: Nihilism
      'Do you feel something terrible has happened or will?'
      'Some people have a feelings that they no longer exist. Have you ever felt like that?'
  Delusions: Persecutory
      'Is anyone trying to harm you?'
      'Is anyone spying on you?'
      'Are there any plots or conspiracies that you know about?'
  Delusions: Reference
      'Do you see any reference to yourself on TV?'
      'Are things ever arranged to have a special meaning?'
  Hallucinations
      'Have you had any odd or unpleasant experiences lately?'
      'Do you ever hear noises or voices when there is nobody about?'
      'Have you ever had visions or seen things other people couldn't?'

Information giving

Description

'We all experience low mood now and then, but the feelings involved in clinical depression are much stronger, more unpleasant and more persistent.'

'Sometimes things can seem so desperate, that people with depression feel that life is not worth living.'

Aetiology

'The cause for depression is not always clear. Sometimes it can follow a stressful life event, but for some people the cause is less obvious.'

Genetics

'A family history of depression increases your risk of becoming depressed. If you have one parent with depression, then you are around eight times more likely to develop depression.'

Personality

'Certain types of personality might mean that you are more likely to become depressed.'

Precipitating factors

'Stressful life events, such as losing one's job can lead people to become depressed.'

Predisposing factors

'Problems during childhood or ongoing difficulties at work or at home can also lead to depression.'

Physical illness

'Some physical illnesses have a strong association with depression. Examples include chronic illnesses such as glandular fever, Parkinson's disease and cardiovascular disease.'

Gender

'Although anyone can become depressed, women are at greater risk than men.'

Prognosis

'Around a quarter of people with depression will recover fully.'

'Around 50–75% will recover, but will experience a further episode in the future.'

'Around a quarter of people with depression will continue to feel depressed for a longer time.'

'With treatment, each episode lasts for around two to three months on average, although for some people, the depression lasts for longer.'

Treatment

Antidepressants

CBT

ECT

Support groups

Depression Alliance

Relate

Samaritans

Essential guidelines (NICE guidelines on depression 2004, amended 2007)

The stepped care model:

Step 1: Recognition (recognising the problem by screening those at risk)

Primary care

Assessment

Step 2: Mild depression

Primary care

Watchful waiting, guided self-help, computerised CBT, brief psychological interventions

Step 3: Moderate or severe depression
  Primary care
  Medication, psychological interventions, social support
Step 4: Treatment-resistant, recurrent, atypical, and psychotic depression and those at significant risk
  Secondary care
  Medication, complex psychological interventions, combined treatments
Step 5: Risk to life, severe self neglect
  Secondary care (usually inpatient)
  Medication, combined treatments, ECT
Secondary care treatment of resistant depression
  Antidepressant + CBT
  Lithium augmentation
  Venlafaxine
  Mirtazepine or mianserin augmentation
  Phenelzine

REFERENCES

Cooper, J. (ed) (2004) *Pocket Guide to the ICD-10: Classification of Mental and Behavioural Disorders*. Churchill Livingstone pp. 131–148

Gelder, M., Harrison, P. & Cowen, P. (2001) *Shorter Oxford Textbook of Psychiatry* (5th edn) Oxford University Press pp. 217–265

Johnstone, EC. & Cunningham Owens, DG. et al. (eds) (2004) *Companion to Psychiatric Studies* (7th edn) . Churchill Livingstone pp. 421–449

NICE Clinical Guidelines: Antenatal and postnatal mental health. National Institute for Clinical Excellence (2004, amended 2007)

Core diagnostic criteria (ICD-10)

Autonomic arousal symptoms
  Palpitations or increased heart rate
  Sweating
  Shaking
  Dry mouth
Symptoms involving chest and abdomen
  Difficulty in breathing
  Feeling of choking
  Chest pain or discomfort
  Nausea or abdominal distress (e.g. churning stomach)
Symptoms involving mental state
  Feeling dizzy, unsteady, faint or light-headed
  Derealization and depersonalization
  Feel of losing control, 'going crazy' or passing out
  Fear of dying
Type of anxiety disorder
  Response to a traumatic specific external stimulus
    Acute stress reaction
    Adjustment disorder
    Post traumatic stress disorder (see separate section)
  Response to a non-traumatic specific external stimulus
    Agoraphobia
    Social phobia
    Specific phobia
  Episodic response to a non-specific external stimulus
    Panic disorder
  Non-episodic response to a non-specific external stimulus
    Generalised anxiety disorder

Key phrases

Confirming symptoms
  'Tell me what happens when you feel anxious.'
  'How often does this happen?'
  'Is there anything you can do to relieve the anxiety?'
  'Would you describe the way you feel as a panic attack?'
Confirming type of anxiety disorder
  'Are you anxious all of the time or only at certain times?'
  'You say that you are anxious all of the time, tell me more about that.'
  'When you feel like this do you ever fear something else might happen?'
  'You say that you only feel anxious at certain times. On these occasions are you anxious for a
  particular reason, such as feeling afraid of leaving the house, or does the feeling just come
  over you?'
Self harm
  'Have you ever felt like harming yourself?'
Co-morbidity
  Depression
  Substance misuse

Obsessive-compulsive disorder
Physical illnesses

Information giving

Management
Medication
Benzodiazepines: can lead to addiction, tolerance and dependence; for short term use only
Antidepressants: a more long term option, up to eight weeks for effect, for minimum six months
Graded exposure therapy with relaxation
'First you will be taught relaxation exercises to control your anxiety and panic. Then you and a therapist will make a list of things that you find difficult to face. Together you will order them from the least difficult to the most difficult. You start by facing the least difficult situation, while managing to relax. When you are comfortable with this we move to the next. You may find it easier to face the situations with the support of a family member or a member of our team.'
Learned controlled breathing
'When we panic we breathe faster to get more oxygen to our muscles to run away or fight. We then breathe out more carbon dioxide and the level of this gas in our blood drops below normal. This causes strange physical sensations like dizziness, breathlessness and tingling in our hands and feet. This is unpleasant and we panic more and breathe even faster. It's a vicious circle. Learning controlled breathing techniques can help to stop this from happening. Some people breathe into a paper bag or cupped hands.'
Cognitive behavioural techniques
See information on cognitive behaviour therapy (CBT)
Family input
'Your family has an important role in helping you. We will teach them about the therapy too so that they can support you.'
Prognosis
'You may not get completely better but many people see great improvements. The outcome is better for people who have good family support and less stress in their life.'
Psychoeducation

Essential guidelines (NICE guidelines on anxiety 2004, amended 2007)

A stepped approach is suggested.
Panic disorder
Not for benzodiazepines
CBT → SSRIs → self-help
Generalised anxiety disorder
Benzodiazepines for two to four weeks only
CBT → SSRIs → self-help

REFERENCES

Cooper, J. (ed) (2004). *Pocket Guide to the ICD-10: Classification of Mental and Behavioural Disorders*. Churchill Livingstone pp. 149–162

Gelder, M., Harrison, P. & Cowen, P. (2001) *Shorter Oxford Textbook of Psychiatry* (5th edn) Oxford University Press pp. 175–201

Johnstone, E.C. & Cunningham Owens, D.G. *et al.* (eds) (2004) *Companion to Psychiatric Studies* (7th edn) Churchill Livingstone pp. 450–485

NICE Clinical Guidelines: Anxiety management of anxiety (panic disorder, with or without agoraphobia, and generalised anxiety disorder) in adults in primary, secondary and community care. National Institute for Clinical Excellence (2004, amended 2007)

OBSESSIVE—COMPULSIVE DISORDER (OCD)

Core diagnostic criteria (ICD-10)

Recurrent obsessional thoughts or compulsive acts
- Obsessional thoughts (ideas, images or impulses that enter the mind)
  - Distressing
  - Thoughts are recognised as patient's own even though they are involuntary and repugnant
- Compulsive acts or rituals (they are repeated again)
  - Not enjoyable but may bring about relief
  - Behaviour is usually recognised as pointless by patient
- Patient often tries unsuccessfully to resist these thoughts and acts
- Causes distress or impairs functioning

Key phrases

Obsessions
  'Let me ask you more about these thoughts. Do they keep coming back to you even when you try not to have them?'
  'Do you find them intrusive?'
  'How do they make you feel in yourself?'
  'Are they distressing?'
Compulsion
  'Do you find you are compelled to do things in a certain way? For example, some people tell themselves they must get up from a chair in a certain way.'
  'What would happen if you tried to resist the need to do things like that?'
  'Have you ever tried?'
  'What happened?'
  'By carrying the compulsion through do you feel a sense of relief?'
  'Do you do things to avoid coming in to contact with dirt or germs?'
  'Do you washing or shower excessively?'
  'Are you always cleaning your house?'
  'Do you repeatedly check things such as whether the oven is turned off?'
  'Do you have to say or read things in certain way?'
Symptom severity
  'How hard do you try to resist these thoughts/actions?'
  'How much control do you have?'
  'How does it affect your day-to-day life?'
Insight
  'Do you think these thoughts/actions are unreasonable?'
  'Do these thoughts come from your own mind?'
  'What would happen if you didn't wash?'
Onset and course
  'When did it all start?'
  'Can you think of any triggers?'
Screen for other dimensions:
  Contamination
    See above
  Order
    'Must things be in certain orders or positions?'
  Aggression
    'Do you fear you may harm others?'

Sexual
    'Do you have any forbidden or seemingly perverse sexual thoughts?'
Religious
    'Are you very concerned with what is right or wrong or blasphemy?'
Confessing
    'Do you have any need to tell or confess?'
Hoarding/collecting
    'Do you have trouble throwing things away?'
Superstition
    'Are you a superstitious person?'
Screen for obsessive—compulsive spectrum disorders
    Body dysmorphic disorder/hypochondriasis
        'Do you have concerns about your body shape or health?'
    Tourette's
        'Have you had any sudden movements or made sounds you were unable to control?'
    Trichotillomania
        'Have you ever purposefully pulled out your hair?'
    Stereotypic movement disorder
        'Do you repeatedly carry out any behaviours such as nail biting, scratching or body rocking?'
Co-morbidity
    Substance misuse
    Psychosis
    Depressive disorder
    Anxiety disorder
    Eating disorder
    Head injury
    Seizure disorder

Information giving

Explain diagnosis
    'It is likely that you have obsessive—compulsive disorder (OCD). People who have this disorder experience similar symptoms to you.'
    'The unwanted and distressing thoughts you described are called obsessions. The actions you told me about, such as how you must check the iron is turned off over and over again, are called compulsions, because you feel compelled to do them. They are also called rituals because they are repeated as if part of a ritual.'
    'It affects two to three people in every 100 during their lifetime. It can be very disabling as you have described.'
Explain treatment
    'It is normal for people with OCD to feel anxious when they do not carry out their rituals. However therapists believe that by challenging the compulsion to carry out rituals, people with OCD can learn to break an ongoing and distressing cycle. Whilst this requires effort on your part, a therapist will be there to help you. The name of the therapy is exposure and response prevention therapy or ERP for short.'
    ERP – the basic principle
        Compulsion = checking lights
        Fear = lights left on
        Escape response = check lights are off
        Exposure = leave lights on
        Outcome = By not checking, the person sees that nothing bad happens

Medication
See below

Essential guidelines (NICE guidelines on obsessive—compulsive disorder 2005)

Mild functional impairment
Brief individual CBT (including ERP)
Moderate functional impairment
SSRI or more intensive CBT (including ERP)
Severe functional impairment
SSRI + CBT (including ERP)
If response is inadequate try a different SSRI or clomipramine
If still no response consider adding antipsychotic or combining SSRI + clomipramine

REFERENCES

Cooper, J. (ed) (2004) *Pocket Guide to the ICD-10: Classification of Mental and Behavioural Disorders.* Churchill Livingstone pp. 162–164
Gelder, M., Harrison, P. & Cowen, P. (2001) *Shorter Oxford Textbook of Psychiatry.* (5th edn) Oxford University Press pp. 175–201
Johnstone, E.C. & Cunningham Owens, D.G. et al. (eds) (2004) *Companion to Psychiatric Studies* (7th edn) Churchill Livingstone pp. 450–485
NICE Clinical Guidelines: Obsessive—compulsive disorder. National Institute for Clinical Excellence (2005)

POSTTRAUMATIC STRESS DISORDER (PTSD)

Core diagnostic criteria (ICD-10)

Delayed or protracted response to a stressful event of a catastrophic nature
Reliving of trauma through
    Intrusive memories (flashbacks)
    Dreams or nightmares
Avoidance of activities and situations reminiscent of trauma
Autonomic hyperarousal
    Insomnia
    Irritability or outbursts of anger
    Difficulties in concentrating
    Hypervigilance
    Exaggerated startle reaction
Emotional blunting or numbness
    Detachment from other people
    Anhedonia

Key phrases

The trauma
    'Do you mind telling me what happened?'
    'Do you remember it clearly?'
    'Were you hurt as a result?'
        'Did you injure your head?'
Reliving of trauma
    'How often do you think about what happened?'
    'Do these memories force their way into your mind?'
    'Do you ever feel like you are reliving what happened?'
    'Do you ever dream or have nightmares about what happened?'
    'Does this ever make you panic?'
        'What happens when you panic?'
        'Does your heart race?'
        'Do you ever feel yourself becoming sweaty or shaky?'
Avoidance of activities and situations reminiscent of trauma
    'Do you deliberately try to avoid thinking about what happened?'
    'Do you ever find yourself avoiding things that remind you of it?'
Autonomic hyperarousal
    'Tell me about your sleep.'
    'Do you lose your temper easily?'
    'How is your concentration?'
    'Do you feel on edge all the time?'
    'Do you startle easily?'
Emotional blunting or numbness
    'Have there been any changes in your feelings generally?'
    'How hard is it for you to talk about these things?'
    'Do you feel numb?'
Distress, impaired social functioning
    'How has all this been affecting you?'
    'Have others commented that you have changed in any way?'
    'How do you spend your time?'
    'How do you feel in yourself generally?'

'How is your family life?'

'How are you getting on at work?'

'Are you socialising as you used to?'

Pre-morbid personality

'Before all of this happened what sort of person were you?'

'How did you previously cope with stress?'

Co-morbidity

Depressive disorder

Anxiety disorder

Somatization

Substance misuse

Insight and expectations

'What do you think the problem is?'

'What do you think we should do?'

Essential guidelines (NICE guidelines on post-traumatic stress disorder 2005)

Stepped approach

Step 1

Mild symptoms, present for less than 4 weeks

Watchful waiting

Follow-up in 1 month

Step 2

Symptoms present for less than 3 months

Trauma focussed CBT, consider hypnotics and antidepressants

Step 3

Symptoms present for more than 3 months

Trauma focussed CBT or eye movement desensitisation and reprocessing (EMDR)

When discussing trauma appointments should be 90 minutes long.

REFERENCES

Cooper, J. (ed) (2004) *Pocket Guide to the ICD-10: Classification of Mental and Behavioural Disorders.* Churchill Livingstone pp. 167–169

Gelder, M., Harrison, P. & Cowen, P. (2001) *Shorter Oxford Textbook of Psychiatry* (5th edn) Oxford University Press pp. 151–173

Johnstone, E.C. & Cunningham Owens, D.G. et al. (eds) *Companion to Psychiatric Studies* (7th edn) Churchill Livingstone pp. 450–485

NICE Clinical Guidelines: Post-traumatic stress disorder (PTSD) the management of PTSD in adults and children in primary and secondary care. National Institute for Clinical Excellence (2005)

GRIEF

Key phrases

Past psychiatric history (makes abnormal grief more likely)
'Have you ever seen anyone from mental health services before?'

Normal grief reaction

Preoccupation with the deceased
'It must be very difficult for you. Does it feel as if you cannot think about anything else?'

Pining or searching
'Sometimes, when someone loses a loved one, they can find themselves searching for them. Has this ever happened to you?'

Somatic responses (e.g. crying, disturbed sleep and changes in appetite)
'How has your sleep been?'
'Has your appetite been affected?'
'Do you feel tearful all the time?'

Mummification
'Have you sorted through any of his belongings?'
'Do you feel comforted by leaving things as they were before his death?'

Hallucinations or illusions of the deceased (usually auditory)
'Sometimes, people hear the voice of their lost loved one. Has this ever happened to you?'
'Some people actually see the deceased person. Have you experienced this?'

Guilt
'People often feel guilty when someone dies. Have you felt like this?'

Thoughts of self-harm or suicide
'Have you ever felt that life is not worth living since he died?'

Abnormal grief reaction

Time course
'When did you start feeling this way?'

Functioning
'How do you manage on a day to day basis?'
'Do you cook yourself meals?'
'Do you manage to do things that you used to?'

Hallucinations
Hallucinations are more bizarre and varied in abnormal grief

Protracted mummification
The whole house may remain exactly as it was, e.g. the table may be set for the deceased. This behaviour does not lessen with time.

Thoughts of self-harm or suicide
Prolonged ideation is more worrying

Acquiring features or symptoms of the deceased's final illness
'How did they die?'
'Have you ever experienced similar pain?'

Idealised view of the deceased

Extras
Grief can also occur following the loss of a pet or a limb
Abnormal grief is more likely following a sudden death or suicide, if the bereaved person was dependent on the deceased, if there is a past psychiatric history, or if there is an inability to grieve because of dependents, such as children.

Stages of loss
Denial
Anger

Bargaining
Depression
Acceptance

Essential guidelines (NICE guidelines on zolpidem, zaleplon and zopiclone 2004)

For severe insomnia interfering with normal daily life

For short periods only

If one Z medication does not work it is not recommended that another is tried from the same group. This should only happen in the event of side-effects.

REFERENCES

Cooper, J. (ed) (2004) *Pocket Guide to the ICD-10: Classification of Mental and Behavioural Disorders.* Churchill Livingstone pp. 169–172

Gelder, M., Harrison, P. & Cowen, P. (2001) *Shorter Oxford Textbook of Psychiatry.* (5th edn) Oxford University Press pp. 151–173

NICE Clinical Guidelines: Guidance on the use of zaleplon, zolpidem and zopiclone for the short-term management of insomnia. National Institute for Clinical Excellence (2004)

SOMATOFORM AND DISSOCIATIVE (CONVERSION) DISORDERS

Somatoform disorders

Somatisation disorder
Multiple, recurrent, frequently changing physical symptoms
   Minimum of two years duration
   Three or more consultations or sets of investigations
      Many negative investigations
      Possible exploratory surgery
   Disruption of social, interpersonal and family behaviour
   Persistent distress
   Persistent refusal to accept medical reassurance
   Gastrointestinal symptoms
      Abdominal pain
      Nausea
      Feeling bloated or full of gas
      Bad taste in the mouth or coated tongue
      Complaints of vomiting or regurgitation of food
      Complaints of loose bowel movements or of fluid from the anus
   Cardiovascular symptoms
      Breathlessness without exertion
      Chest pains
   Genitourinary symptoms
      Dysuria or complaints of frequency of micturition
      Unpleasant sensations in or around the genitals
      Complaints of unusual or copious vaginal discharge
   Skin and pain symptoms
      Blotchiness or discoloration of the skin
   Pain in the limbs, extremities or joints
   Unpleasant numbness or tingling sensations
Hypochondriacal disorder
   Persistent belief of having one or more serious physical disease
   Minimum six months duration
   Persistent distress
   Interference with personal functioning in daily living
   Seeks medical treatment or investigations
   Persistent refusal to accept medical reassurance
Body dysmorphic disorder (type of hypochondriacal disorder)
   Persistent preoccupation with a presumed body deformity or disfigurement that is non-delusional
   The delusional type is called delusional dysmorphobia

Dissociative (conversion) disorder

There is no evidence of physical cause
There are associations in time between onset and stress
Symptoms often represent the patient's concept of how a physical illness would manifest
Only includes disorders of functions normally under voluntary control and decreased sensation
Types of dissociative disorders
   Dissociative amnesia

Dissociative fugue
   Unexpected journey away, amnesia for the journey
Dissociative stupor
Trance and possession disorder
   Decreased consciousness, feeling of having been taken over
Dissociative motor disorder
   Loss of limb movement
Dissociative convulsions
Dissociative anaesthesia and sensory loss
Ganser's syndrome
   Approximate answers
   Clouded consciousness
   Somatic symptoms
   Pseudohallucinations
Multiple personality disorder

Management

See the same doctor and regularly
SSRIs for body dysmorphic syndrome or if underlying depressive disorder
Some psychotherapy can help, usually CBT (not usually psychoanalytical as insight orientated) or group therapy
Tends to remit after a few weeks or months

REFERENCES

Cooper, J. (ed) (2004) *Pocket Guide to the ICD-10: Classification of Mental and Behavioural Disorders.* Churchill Livingstone pp. 172–192

Gelder, M., Harrison, P. & Cowen, P. (2001) *Shorter Oxford Textbook of Psychiatry* (5th edn) Oxford University Press pp. 203–216

Guthrie, E. & Creed, F. (eds) (2004) *College Seminars Series: Seminars in Liaison Psychiatry* The Royal College of Psychiatrists pp. 103–156

Johnstone, E.C. & Cunningham Owens, D.G. et al. (eds) (2004) *Companion to Psychiatric Studies* (7th edn) Churchill Livingstone pp. 450–485 & 693–696

NEURASTHENIA

Core diagnostic criteria (ICD-10)

Core feature
>   Persistent and distressing complaints of feelings of exhaustion or weakness after minor mental or physical effort
>   The patient is unable to recover from feelings of fatigue by means of rest, relaxation or entertainment

Symptoms
>   Aches and pains
>   Dizziness
>   Tension headaches
>   Sleep disturbance
>   Inability to relax
>   Irritability

Other features
>   Poor concentration
>   Autonomic symptoms (cardiovascular or gastrointestinal)
>   Frequent waking or hypersomnia

Core diagnostic criteria (Oxford Criteria for Chronic Fatigue Syndrome)

This affects both physical and mental functioning
It is present for more than 50% of the time
Exclusion criteria apply

Information giving

What is neurasthenia?
>   'Neurasthenia is the name given to the illness which results in feelings of exhaustion after minor mental or physical effort as you have described today.'
>   'Neurasthenia is also known as chronic fatigue syndrome and ME.'

What causes it?
>   'It may occur following a viral condition or may be part of depressive or nervous illness.'

Treatment
>   Rehabilitation
>   CBT
>   Antidepressants

REFERENCES

Cooper, J. (ed) (2004) *Pocket Guide to the ICD-10: Classification of Mental and Behavioural Disorders* Churchill Livingstone pp. 192–194

Guthrie, E. & Creed, F. (eds) (2004) *College Seminars Series: Seminars in Liaison Psychiatry.* The Royal College of Psychiatrists pp. 103–156

Johnstone, EC. & Cunningham Owens, D.G. *et al.* (ed) (2004) *Companion to Psychiatric Studies* (7th edn) Churchill Livingstone pp. 450–485 & 694

ANOREXIA NERVOSA AND BULIMIA NERVOSA

Anorexia nervosa

Core diagnostic criteria (ICD-10)

Deliberate weight loss
- Self-induced avoidance of fattening foods
- Excessive exercise
- Induced vomiting and purgation
- Use of appetite suppressants and diuretics

Self-perception of being too fat and intrusive dread of being fat
- Leads to a self-imposed low weight threshold

Under nutrition
- Secondary endocrine and metabolic changes with disturbances of bodily function

Key phrases

Deliberate weight loss
- 'Can you tell me what you ate yesterday?'
- 'It sounds like you allow yourself very little food. Is this to lose weight?'
- 'Do you avoid eating certain foods because of your diet?'
    - 'Tell me which foods you avoid.'
- 'Have you ever starved yourself completely?'
- 'How long did that last for?'
- 'Do you do anything else to lose weight such as exercise?'
- 'How much exercise do you do?'
- 'Have you ever made yourself be sick in order to get rid of food that you have eaten?'
- 'Have you ever used laxatives or other preparations in order to weigh less?'
- 'Have you ever used diuretics in order to weigh less?'
- 'Have you ever used diet pills or appetite suppressants?'
    - 'What were they called?'
- 'Do you have diabetes or thyroid disease?'
- 'Have you ever withheld your insulin or you thyroid medication to prevent weight gain?'

Self-perception of being too fat and intrusive dread of being fat
- 'What is your current weight?'
- 'Do you think you are overweight?'
- 'What is your ideal weight?'
- 'How often do you weigh yourself?'
- 'Do you measure yourself?'
- 'Do you find yourself looking in the mirror all of the time?'
- 'How do you feel about yourself?'

Under nutrition
- Endocrine changes
- To women
    - 'How old were you when you had your first period?'
    - 'How often do you have a period?'
    - 'When was your last period?'
    - 'Has there ever been a time when you have not had your period?'
        - Remember that amenorrhoea may be masked by taking the oral contraceptive pill
- To men
    - 'Have you noticed any change in your interest in having sex?'
    - 'Are you having any difficulties in having sexual intercourse?'

Information giving

What is anorexia nervosa?

'Anorexia is a type of eating disorder where people deliberately lose weight because they fear they are overweight. With anorexia it is very difficult for people to see that they are under rather than overweight, and no amount of reassurance will usually convince them otherwise.'

'Anorexia affects about 1 in every 200 people during their lifetime.'

Weight in anorexia nervosa

Body weight < 85% expected, BMI < 17.5

Treatment

Physical

Full physical examination, bloods, ECG, bone density scan

Any drugs should be prescribed with care

Re-feeding: Aim for weight increase of 0.5–1kg per week

Re-feed against will as a last resort

Psychological

CBT

CAT

Interpersonal therapy (IPT)

Focal psychodynamic therapy

Family interventions

Eating diaries

Patient education

Prognosis

'People do recover from anorexia. Scientific studies show that around half of people with anorexia are better after ten years.'

Essential guidelines (NICE guidelines on eating disorders 2004)

Most people should be managed as an outpatient with psychological treatment (see treatment section above)

Medication should not be used as the sole or primary treatment

Feeding against the will of the patient should be an intervention of last resort and the legal basis must be clear

Bulimia nervosa

Core diagnostic criteria (ICD-10)

Recurrent episodes of overeating

Persistent preoccupation with eating and a strong desire to eat (craving)

Excessive preoccupation with the control of body weight

Self-induced vomiting

Self-induced purging

Use of appetite suppressants and diuretics

Self-perception of being too fat and intrusive dread of being fat

Usually leads to being underweight

Key phrases

Recurrent episodes of overeating

'Do you ever find yourself eating lots of food in a short space of time?'

'What would you usually eat during one of these binges?'
'How often do you eat like this?'
'Does anything make you do this?'
'What makes you stop eating?'
'How do you feel afterwards?'
Persistent preoccupation with eating and a strong desire to eat (craving)
'Do you get cravings for food?'
'What sorts of food do you crave?'
'Do you make do with what food you have to hand when you get a craving or do you make a special journey?'
Excessive preoccupation with the control of body weight
See *Deliberate weight loss* in *Anorexia nervosa* section above.
Self-perception of being too fat and intrusive dread of being fat
See *Anorexia nervosa* section above

Information giving

What is bulimia nervosa?
'Bulimia is a type of eating disorder. People with bulimia are excessively preoccupied with their weight and dread being fat. Alongside this fear is the desire to binge on large amounts of food. However, this leads to self-loathing and people with bulimia often resort to making themselves sick immediately afterwards to prevent weight gain.'
'Bulimia affects about 2 in every 100 people during their lifetime.'
Weight in bulimia nervosa
May be underweight or overweight
Treatment
Physical
SSRI (typically fluoxetine 60mg)
Psychological
See *Anorexia nervosa* section above for further details

Essential guidelines (NICE guidelines on eating disorders 2004)

Step 1
Patients should be encouraged to follow an evidenced-based self help programme in the first instance and/or an antidepressant drug
Step 2
Cognitive behaviour therapy for bulimia nervosa (CBT-BN), a specifically adapted form of CBT should be offered

REFERENCES
Cooper, J. (ed) (2004) *Pocket Guide to the ICD-10: Classification of Mental and Behavioural Disorders.* Churchill Livingstone pp. 197–200
Gelder, M., Harrison, P. & Cowen, P. (2001) *Shorter Oxford Textbook of Psychiatry* (5th edn) Oxford University Press pp. 259–371
Johnstone, E.C. & Cunningham Owens, D.G. et al. (eds) (2004) *Companion to Psychiatric Studies* (7th edn) Churchill Livingstone pp. 486–501
NICE Clinical Guidelines: Core interventions in the treatment and management of anorexia nervosa, bulimia nervosa and related eating disorders. (2004) National Institute for Clinical Excellence

POSTNATAL BLUES, DEPRESSION AND PSYCHOSIS

Postnatal blues

Features
   Tearfulness, low mood, emotional lability and confusion
Onset
   Usually a few days after delivery
Course
   Usually resolves in a few days
Epidemiology
   Up to half of mothers are affected

Postnatal depression

Features
   Similar to depressive episode
   Onset
   Usually within 3 months of delivery
Course
   Similar to depressive episode
   Epidemiology
   10–15% of mothers are affected
Screening for postnatal depression
   See diagnostic criteria for *Depressive disorder*
Management of postnatal depression
   Counselling, self-help groups, psychotherapy
   Antidepressants
   Admission to mother and baby unit
   ECT in certain circumstances

Puerperal psychosis

Features
   Hallucinations, delusions, perplexity, restlessness, anxiety, mania (affective psychosis is most common), severe insomnia in the absence of the baby crying
Onset
   Abrupt (0.2% of mothers of live births are affected)
Management of puerperal psychosis
   Admission to mother and baby unit
   Lithium if psychosis is affective
   Antipsychotic medication
   Antidepressants
   Supportive counselling
   Psychotherapy
   ECT
Consider risk to mother and baby
   Suicide
   Harm to baby
   Harm to others

Essential guidelines (NICE guidelines on antenatal and postnatal mental health 2004)

At first contact with services in both the antenatal and postnatal periods, healthcare professionals should ask about psychiatric history and family history or perinatal mental illness. There should be quick access to psychological therapies (one to three months).

Contraception and the risks associated with pregnancy in mental illness (including relapse, risks associated with stopping or changing medication and risk to the foetus) should be discussed with all women of child-bearing potential.

REFERENCES

Cooper, J. (ed) (2004) *Pocket Guide to the ICD-10: Classification of Mental and Behavioural Disorders* Churchill Livingstone pp. 216–217

Gelder, M., Harrison, P. & Cowen, P. (2001) *Shorter Oxford Textbook of Psychiatry* (5th edn) Oxford University Press pp. 402–403

Johnstone, E.C. & Cunningham Owens, D.G. *et al.* (eds) (2004) *Companion to Psychiatric Studies* (7th edn) Churchill Livingstone pp. 741–753.

NICE Clinical Guidelines: Antenatal and postnatal mental health (2004) National Institute for Clinical Excellence

Core diagnostic criteria (ICD-10)

Impulsive type = three impulsive traits
Borderline = three impulsive + three borderline traits
Impulsive
- (S) Sudden mood changes
- (Q) Quarrelsome
- (U) Unpredictable acts (no thought of consequences)
- (A) Angry and violent towards others
- (D) Difficulty in maintaining action with no immediate reward

Borderline
- (S) Self image disturbance
- (H) Harm to self (or threats to harm self)
- (A) Abandonment avoidance efforts
- (R) Relationships are unstable and intense
- (E) Emptiness feelings

Key phrases

Sudden mood changes
'How is your mood?'
'Does your mood change frequently?'
Quarrelsome
'Do you find yourself arguing with people a lot of the time?'
'Do people ever criticise your behaviour?'
'How does this make you feel?'
Unpredictable acts
'Do you ever do things on the spur of the moment and then regret them?'
'Do you like taking risks?'
'Do you drive?'
'Would you say you are a safe driver or do you like risking it?'
'Do you ever stop to think what might happen when you decide to do something?'
Angry and violent towards others
'Do you think you could have a problem with your temper?'
'Does your temper get you into fights?'
'Do you find it hard to calm down once you have lost your temper?'
Risk of harm to others
'Have you ever harmed anyone else?'
'Have you ever been in trouble with the law?'
'Is there anyone you wish to come to harm?'
Difficulty in maintaining action with no immediate reward
'Do you find it hard to stick at something which does not offer a quick reward?'
Self image disturbance (goals, plans in work, friendships, romantic life)
'Do you feel that your goals often change?'
'Has this made your life difficult in any way?'
Harm to self (or threats to harm self)
'Do you self-harm?'
'Do you do this regularly?'
Efforts to avoid abandonment
'How often do you feel abandoned or left to cope on your own?'
'How do you react when you feel this way?'

Unstable and intense relationships
    'How have your relationships worked out for you?'
    'How many serious relationships have you had?'
Chronic feelings of emptiness
    'Do you often feel as if you are empty inside?'
    'Do you ever feel as though life is meaningless?'
    'Do you get bored easily?'
Transient paranoid symptoms
    Elicit delusional ideas
Transient dissociative symptoms
    'Do you ever feel unreal or cut off like a zombie?'
    'Have you ever had periods in your day or week that you can't account for?'
Co-morbidity
    Depressive disorder
    Anxiety disorder
    Panic disorder
    Substance misuse
    Eating disorder
    Psychosis
    Post-traumatic stress disorder
Past history
    Early abuse (physical, sexual, emotional and neglect)
    Emotional inconsistency and unpredictable care giving
    Bullying and difficulties at school

Information giving

What is borderline personality disorder?
    'It is likely that you have something called borderline personality disorder. Your early
    experiences may have left you with problems in calming yourself down, relating to people
    and in feeling confident about who you are. You may feel intense emotions that change
    quickly. You may have made impulsive decisions, which turned out badly.'
Treatment
    Psychotherapy (especially DBT)
    Medication - modest benefits are seen with
        Conventional antipsychotics
        SSRIs (to reduce impulsivity and aggression)
        Mood stabilizers

REFERENCES

Cooper, J. (ed) (2004) *Pocket Guide to the ICD-10: Classification of Mental and Behavioural Disorders* Churchill Livingstone pp. 228–229

Gelder, M, Harrison, P. & Cowen, P. (2001) *Shorter Oxford Textbook of Psychiatry* (5th edn) Oxford University Press pp. 127–150

NICE Clinical Guidelines (2009) *Borderline Personality Disorder.* National Institute for Clinical Excellence.

Johnstone, E.C. & Cunningham Owens, D.G. *et al.* (eds) *Companion to Psychiatric Studies* (7th edn) Churchill Livingstone pp. 502–526

Taylor, D., Paton, C. & Kerwin, R. (2007) *The South London and Maudsley NHS Foundation Trust & Oxleas NHS Foundation Trust Prescribing Guidelines* (9th edn) Informa Healthcare pp. 462–464

Key phrases

Details of seizures

'What happens when you have a seizure?'

'Has anyone seen you having a seizure?'

'What do they say happens?'

'How long have you been having seizures for?'

'How often do they happen?'

'How long does each one last?'

'How do they affect your daily life?'

'Do they stop you doing certain things?'

Medication history

'Do you take any medications?'

Pay particular attention to psychotropic medications which are known to lower the seizure threshold.

'Do the seizures happen at a certain time after taking the medication?'

'Do you think that the medication is making your seizures happen more frequently?'

'Has the dose ever been changed?'

'What affect has this change had on your seizures?'

Family history

'Has anyone in your family ever had a seizure?'

'Have they been diagnosed with epilepsy?'

Past medical history

'Have you ever had a head injury?'

'Do you have any other health problems?'

'Do you drink alcohol?'

'Have you ever had a fit whilst running a fever?'

Screening for associated psychosis

'Have you ever experienced bizarre thoughts or seen things other people haven't inbetween your seizures?'

Auras

'Some people experience auras before a seizure; in other words they experience a strange sensation. Examples of such sensations include experiencing an unpleasant smell. Has anything like that ever happened to you?'

'Can you tell me more about what happens?'

Déjà vu

'Other people feel that they are living a new experience which seems so familiar that it feels like they have lived it before. People call this déjà vu. Has this ever happened to you?'

Jamais vu

'Other people have an eerie sense that a situation they know they recognise feels new to them. Has this ever happened to you?'

Information giving

Management of the epilepsy

Medication

Anti-epileptic drugs (see *Essential guidelines* below)

Responsibility of care

Diagnosis and ongoing management decisions should be made by a specialist

An epilepsy specialist nurse should be an integral part of care

Support groups
Epilepsy Action
Management of associated psychosis
Antipsychotic medication

Essential guidelines (NICE guidelines on epilepsy 2004)

First-line anti-epileptic drugs for focal epilepsies include carbamazepine, lamotrigine, oxcarbazepine, sodium valproate and topiramate.
Individuals should be treated with a single anti-epileptic drug where possible.
A referral to tertiary services should be considered where there is a psychiatric comorbidity.

REFERENCES

NICE Clinical Guidelines: Epilepsy in Adults and Children (2004) National Institute for Clinical Excellence

Joint Formulary Committee. British National Formulary (56th edn) (2008) British Medical Association and Royal Pharmaceutical Society of Great Britain pp. 246–258

King, D.J. (ed) (2004) *College Seminars Series: Seminars in Clinical Psychopharmacology* (2nd edn) The Royal College of Psychiatrists pp. 381–412

Warrell, D.A., Cox, T.M., Firth, J.D. & Benz, E.J. (ed) (2006) *Oxford Textbook of Medicine* (4th edn) Oxford University Press

EXTRA PYRAMIDAL SIDE EFFECTS (EPSEs)

Key phrases

Drug history
    'What medication do you take?'
    'What dose are you on?'
    'How long have you been taking this medication?'
    'Has your dose been changed recently?'
Symptom history
    Akathisia
        'Have you had any feelings of restlessness in your legs?'
        'Do you feel you need to pace up and down?'
    Bradykinesia
        'Have you felt as if you've been slowed down?'
    Tardive dyskinesia
        'Have you had any unusual or uncomfortable movements of the face?'
        'Have your family or friends ever noticed anything?'
    Stiffness
        'Have your muscles ever felt stiff?'
    Spasms
        'Do you ever get muscle spasms?'
    Shakiness
        'Do your hands ever feel shaky?'
        'Do you ever spill drinks?'
        Men only
        'Do you ever have trouble shaving?'
    Hypersalivation
        'Do you ever feel as if you have to swallow more saliva?'
        'Does your pillow feel wet in the morning?'
    Dystonia

Examination

Hands and upper limbs when sitting
    Akathisia
        Hands on thighs with palms down
    Tremor
        Hands and arms stretched out
        Balance paper on outstretched hands
    Bradykinesia
        Opposition of thumb with each finger, one by one
        'Raise your arms to your shoulder height and then let them fall to your sides, like me'
        [demonstrate]
    Tone
        Clasp-knife
        Cogwheeling
    Reflexes
Mouth when sitting
    Inspect mouth, checking for tremors, dystonia, and tardive dyskinesia
    Repeat above with tongue protruded
Standing - inspection, looking for dystonia of trunk muscles

Gait
   Is the gait festinant?
   Is there unsteadiness?

REFERENCES

Douglas, G., Nicol, F. & Robertson, C. (2005) *Macleod's Clinical Examination* (11th edn) Churchill Livingstone

Gelder, M., Harrison, P. & Cowen, P. (2001) *Shorter Oxford Textbook of Psychiatry* (5th edn) Oxford University Press pp. 534–540

NEUROLEPTIC MALIGNANT SYNDROME AND SEROTONIN SYNDROME

Neuroleptic malignant syndrome (NMS)

Core information

Incidence around 1%

Mortality up to 20%

Forty per cent get medical complications

Associated with high potency antipsychotics (usually typicals)

Occurs hours to months after initial exposure, typically within days

Essential features
- Fever (may be mild)
- Altered consciousness (especially delirium)
- Autonomic instability
    - Tachycardia
    - Unstable or labile blood pressure
    - Diaphoresis (profuse sweating)
    - Pallor/flushing
    - Increased respiratory rate
- Muscular rigidity (usually 'leadpipe', not relieved by anticholinergics)

Other features
- Sialorrhoea (excessive secretion of saliva)
- Akinesia
- Bradykinesia
- Dyskinesia
- Mutism
- Dysphasia
- Dysarthria
- Dysphagia
- Ataxia
- Nystagmus
- Seizures
- Incontinence

Laboratory findings
- Grossly elevated creatinine phosphokinase (CPK)
- Leucocytosis
- Hyperkalaemia
- Hypomagnesaemia
- Anaemia
- Increased erythrocyte sedimentation rate (ESR)
- Proteinuria
- Myoglobuminuria
- EEG excessive slow waves

Risk factors
- Male
- Organic brain disease
- Physical exhaustion
- Dehydration
- Affective disorders
- Neuroleptic naivety

Assessment
- Vital signs (temperature, blood pressure, heart rate, respiratory rate)
- Physical examination including neurological observations
- Mental state examination
- Laboratory investigations (including urgent CPK, U&Es, FBC, urine sample)

Essential guidelines (Maudsley guidelines 2007)

Management of neuroleptic malignant syndrome
- In the psychiatric unit
  - Withdraw antipsychotics
  - Monitor temperature, pulse and blood pressure
  - Involve medical colleagues urgently
- In the medical/A&E unit
  - Rehydration
  - Bromocriptine (dopamine agonist)
  - Dantrolene (muscle relaxant)
  - Sedation with benzodiazepines
  - Artificial ventilation if required
  - Consider ECT for treatment of psychosis
- Restarting antipsychotics
  - Antipsychotic rechallenge will be required in most instances
  - Stop antipsychotics for at least five days
  - Begin rechallenge with very small dose and increase slowly
  - Close monitoring of physical and biochemical parameters is essential

Serotonin syndrome

Core information

This is caused by administering two antidepressants simultaneously, usually by combining monoamine-oxidase inhibitors (MAOIs) with serotonin augmenters (SSRIs, trazodone or tricyclics).

Clinical features
- Ataxia*
- Altered mental state*
- Delirium*
- Fever*
- Rigors
- Seizures*
- Diaphoresis*
- Myoclonus
- Tremor
- Restlessness
- Hyperreflexia
- Hypomania
- Shivering/chattering teeth
- Diarrhoea
- Incoordination
- Potentially fatal
- (* = also possible with NMS)

Management of serotonin syndrome
> Stop all medication
> Give supportive treatment

Essential guidelines (Maudsley guidelines 2007)

How to avoid serotonin syndrome
> Cross-taper antidepressants with caution
> Ensure week wash out period for all MAOIs

REFERENCES

Gelder, M., Harrison, P. & Cowen, P. (2001) *Shorter Oxford Textbook of Psychiatry.* (5th edn) Oxford University Press pp. 536–551

Johnstone, E.C. & Cunningham Owens, D.G. *et al.* (eds) (2004) *Companion to Psychiatric Studies* (7th edn) Churchill Livingstone p. 267

King, D.J. (ed). *College Seminars Series: Seminars in Clinical Psychopharmacology* (2nd edn) (2004) The Royal College of Psychiatrists pp. 221–223

Taylor, D., Paton, C. & Kerwin, R. (2007) *The South London and Maudsley NHS Foundation Trust & Oxleas NHS Foundation Trust Prescribing Guidelines* (9th edn) Informa Healthcare (pp. 103–105)

ANTIDEPRESSANTS

Information giving

Do antidepressants work?

'Seven out of ten people will get better on antidepressant medication. Other things which help include having someone to talk to, taking regular exercise, not drinking alcohol in excess, eating well and using self help techniques to relax.'

How do they work?

'When people are depressed some of the chemicals in the brain do not work properly.'

'Antidepressants can normalise these chemicals and help us to feel better.'

How long does it take?

'It usually takes between two and eight weeks for the medications to have their full effect.'

'We suggest that the minimum time to continue taking them is six months after you feel better. Some people may need to continue taking them for longer than this to stay well. It is important to take the medication every day for it to work properly.'

What else are they used for?

'Antidepressants are also used for anxiety, panic attacks, obsessions, chronic pain, eating disorders and post traumatic stress syndrome.'

What about getting pregnant?

'It is in the first three months of pregnancy that the mother's medication affects the baby the most. We try to avoid all medication during this time. However, we have to weigh up the pros and cons. If you do need to have antidepressants during this time it may be better to have one of the older antidepressants. The risk in breast feeding is very small.'

Are they addictive?

'Antidepressants are not addictive.'

'They do not cause tolerance or craving.'

'They will not make you feel like a zombie.'

Stopping antidepressants

'It is often best to stop taking the medication gradually, reducing the dose over a few weeks. This helps to reduce any side effects of discontinuation like headaches, flu-like symptoms and strange neurological symptoms such as electricity-like sensations.'

Side effects

'Some side effects may be present initially. These are usually mild and stop after the first few weeks. Side effects may include dry mouth, blurred vision, constipation, diarrhoea, nausea, erectile dysfunction, loss of sex drive or problems achieving orgasm. If any of these problems persist we can consider changing the dose of the medication or trying a different drug.'

Offer to provide written information

Refer to resources sheet

Essential guidelines (NICE Depression 2004)

Antidepressants are not recommended for the initial treatment of mild depression unless there is a history of moderate or severe depression because the risk-benefit ratio is poor.

For routine care, use an SSRI because they are as effective as tricyclic antidepressants and are less likely to be discontinued because of side effects.

REFERENCES

Gelder, M., Harrison, P. & Cowen, P. (2001) *Shorter Oxford Textbook of Psychiatry* (5th edn) Oxford University Press pp. 540–557

Johnstone, E.C. & Cunningham Owens, D.G. et al. (eds) (2004) *Companion to Psychiatric Studies* (7th edn) Churchill Livingstone pp. 271–285 & 438–439

(56th edn) (2008)British Medical Association and Royal Pharmaceutical Society of Great Britain pp. 204–215

King, D.J. (ed) (2004) College Seminars Series: Seminars in Clinical Psychopharmacology (2nd edn) The Royal College of Psychiatrists pp. 178–243

NICE Clinical Guidelines: Depression management of depression in primary and secondary care (2004) National Institute for Clinical Excellence (2004)

LITHIUM

Information giving

Indications

'Lithium is used for a number of conditions, including bipolar affective disorder, but also mania, hypomania and recurrent depression.'

'It is a tried and tested medication that has been used for many years.'

'It is usually considered when there have been two periods of illness in two years or three periods of illness in five years.'

'It is also a good choice when other mood stabilizers have not worked.'

Tolerance and monitoring

'Lithium is not the easiest of medications to take. The reasons for this are the side effects and the blood tests.'

'However, if you are OK with the blood tests and can tolerate mild side effects, if you get them, then you will probably get on OK with lithium.'

'We require regular blood tests to monitor the levels of the drug in your blood and to keep an eye on your kidney and thyroid function, as lithium can affect them both.'

'Lithium levels need to be kept within a certain range. If the levels are too low the drug is not effective and if they are too high they can cause toxicity.'

'Lithium can cause the thyroid to become under active and can cause kidney function to deteriorate.'

'We also need an ECG, or heart tracing, before we commence treatment.'

Side effects

'Common side effects include: stomach cramps, diarrhoea, tremor and mild thirst; others include passing large volumes of urine and passing urine more frequently, and weight gain.'

Dehydration

'Causes of dehydration, such as vomiting, diarrhoea or indeed prolonged periods of exercise, can increase the blood lithium levels, which can lead to lithium toxicity. You would need to ensure that you always drink enough water.'

Contraindications

Renal impairment

Thyroid disease

Cardiac disease

Sodium imbalance, e.g. in Addison's disease

Drug interactions

Diuretics

Non steroidal anti-inflammatory drugs (NSAIDS)

Lithium and travel

Information giving

Before the trip

'Travelling puts strain on those with bipolar affective disorder'

'Before long-distance travel, it is best that you reduce as many unnecessary activities as possible and only do the essentials.'

'Travel can cause a lot of stress due to excitement before leaving, the physical stress of flying and changes in the environment. It is important that you keep to your routine in the days leading up to your trip.'

'Anticipation and excitement can cause problems with sleep. Short-term benzodiazepines, such as diazepam, may be of use to you leading up to your trip.'

'Relaxation techniques before bed can also help.'

Medical declaration

'I can give you a letter to take with you when travelling so that if you need treatment when you're holiday so that the doctors and nurses will know what treatment you're on at home.'

Travelling and destination

'Make sure you drink plenty of fluids and avoid alcohol.'

'If you're going somewhere hot, remember that you may become dehydrated very quickly and this may lead to dangerous levels of lithium in your blood.'

'Vomiting, diarrhoea and fever can all lead to dehydration so it would be a good idea if you took remedies for these with you.'

Further suggestions

'Comprehensive travel insurance including health cover is vital.'

'It's a good idea to split your medication between your suitcase and your hand luggage in case of lost baggage.'

'Pack extra medication in case your flight is delayed.'

'Remember to take your lithium card, which will help remind you of the signs of lithium toxicity.'

'You may also want to consider wearing a medical alert bracelet.'

Lithium and hypothyroidism

Information giving

'We monitor thyroid function regularly, as there is a risk that lithium can interfere with the thyroid gland.'

'It's nothing to be too worried about, but it is something we will need to monitor and correct.'

'The thyroid gland produces hormones necessary for bodily function, in particular metabolism. In hypothyroidism, the hormone levels are low due to underproduction of the hormones by the gland. This occurs in 1 in 20 people taking lithium.'

'The condition normally comes on slowly, so you may not have noticed any symptoms. I have noticed from your blood results that your levels of thyroid hormones are low. The good news is that the condition can be treated effectively by replacing the hormone in the form of a tablet called levothyroxine.'

Clinical symptoms of hypothyroidism

Lack of energy

Cold intolerance

Slowness in thought and action

Hoarseness

Weight gain

Changes in hair and skin texture

Pins and needles

Constipation

Mood (particularly depression)

Thyroid examination

Ask permission

Inspection

Ask patient to expose their neck

Make a show of looking at the thyroid from the front

Look at the eyes from the sides and from above

Ask patient to take some water into the mouth and hold it there

Make a show of watching the thyroid as they swallow

Palpation
    Ask permission to feel patient's neck
    Stand behind and to the right
    Feel the left and right lobes with both hands
    Ask them to swallow water whilst palpating
    Examine local lymph nodes
Percussion
Auscultation
    Listen to both lobes of the thyroid for bruits and then the chest for arrhythmias
Investigations
    Ultrasound of neck and thyroid (a CT or MRI may also be needed)
    Radioactive thyroid scan
    Fine needle aspiration biopsy (FNAB)
    Chest X-ray

Essential guidelines (NICE guidelines on bipolar disorder 2006)

Continue trial of lithium for at least six months to establish effectiveness.

Aim for 0.6–0.8mmol/l or 0.9–1.0mmol/l if the patient has previously relapsed whilst taking lithium.

If lithium is stopped or is about to be stopped abruptly, consider changing to an atypical antipsychotic and monitor for early signs of mania and depression.

REFERENCES

Douglas, G., Nicol, F. & Robertson, C. (2005) *Macleod's Clinical Examination* (11th edn) Churchill Livingstone

Gelder, M., Harrison, P. & Cowen, P. (2001) *Shorter Oxford Textbook of Psychiatry* (5th edn) Oxford University Press pp. 557–561

Joint Formulary Committee. British National Formulary (56th edn) (2008) British Medical Association and Royal Pharmaceutical Society of Great Britain pp. 202–204

King, D.J. (ed) (2004) *College Seminars Series: Seminars in Clinical Psychopharmacology* (2nd edn) The Royal College of Psychiatrists pp. 244–279

NICE Clinical Guidelines: Bipolar disorder the management of bipolar disorder in adults, children and adolescents, in primary and secondary care. (2006) National Institute for Clinical Excellence

Taylor, D., Paton, C. & Kerwin, R. (2007) *The South London and Maudsley NHS Foundation Trust & Oxleas NHS Foundation Trust Prescribing Guidelines* (9th edn) Informa Healthcare pp. 147–152

CLOZAPINE

Information giving

Rationale

'Clozapine is mainly used in treatment resistant schizophrenia and it is a very effective medication'

Side effects

'As with every medication there are side effects with clozapine. Some are common and some are rare.'

'Many of the side effects should wear off after three to four weeks.'

'Common side effects include: sedation, an increase or a decrease in blood pressure, fever, nausea, constipation and excess saliva production.'

'Many of the side effects can be treated easily. For example patients who become constipated may need to start taking a gentle laxative.'

'It can also cause weight gain, although we will help you watch this and we can give you dietary advice.'

'The most serious side-effect is a drop in the white blood cells, which are responsible for fighting infection. However this is very rare.'

'It only happens to between one and three people in every 100. As a precaution we monitor the levels of these blood cells in people taking clozapine by taking blood samples.'

'Blood samples are collected weekly for the first 18 weeks, then fortnightly until 52 weeks, and then monthly thereafter.'

'To make sure this monitoring goes smoothly, every patient taking clozapine has to be registered with a clozapine patient management service.'

'When we take these blood samples we may also check the level of clozapine in your blood at the same time. This is to make sure you are taking the correct dose for you and not too much or too little.'

'There is also a slight risk of inflammation of the heart muscle, which is called myocarditis. We will perform an ECG before starting clozapine for this reason.'

If the patient is put off by the number of side-effects

'Of course not everyone gets all of the side effects, but I think that it's important to tell you about these things.'

'Clozapine is a very effective drug and you will be monitored very closely.'

'Another benefit of clozapine is that it is less likely to cause tremor and unwanted movements than you can get with other medications'

Commencing clozapine

'Ideally, we like to start clozapine in hospital at first, but we could also do this from home with close monitoring.'

If the patient says that he does not want clozapine

'Why don't you have a think about it and we can meet again.'

'Perhaps you would like to talk to your friends or family or some patients who take clozapine and see what they have to say.'

Interactions

Smoking

'Smoking can lead to a reduction in clozapine levels by as much as half so it is especially important that we monitor Clozapine levels in smokers.'

Caffeine

'Clozapine levels may be increased by caffeine which is contained in tea, coffee and chocolate.'

Other medication

'It can also interact with other medications so we need to monitor what you are taking and how much.'

Epilepsy

'In people who have epilepsy, clozapine can increase the risk of having a seizure.'

Clozapine augmentation

'In rare cases Clozapine only is not enough to control the symptoms. If this happens we could consider adding in another medication to work alongside the Clozapine.'

Essential guidelines (NICE guidelines on schizophrenia 2002)

Clozapine should be considered if there is no significant improvement after two antipsychotics (including one atypical) have each been used for six to eight weeks.

REFERENCES

Gelder, M., Harrison, P. & Cowen, P. (2001) *Shorter Oxford Textbook of Psychiatry* (5th edn Oxford University Press pp. 532–536

Johnstone, E.C. & Cunningham Owens, D.G. et al. (ed) (2004) *Companion to Psychiatric Studies*(7th edn) Churchill Livingstone pp. 257–269

Joint Formulary Committee. British National Formulary (56th edn) (2008) British Medical Association and Royal Pharmaceutical Society of Great Britain pp. 197–198

King, D.J. (ed) *College Seminars Series: Seminars in Clinical Psychopharmacology* (2nd edn) (2004) The Royal College of Psychiatrists pp. 316–380

NICE Clinical Guidelines: Schizophrenia core interventions in the treatment and management of schizophrenia in primary and secondary care (2002) National Institute for Clinical Excellence

Taylor, D., Paton, C. & Kerwin, R. (2007) *The South London and Maudsley NHS Foundation Trust & Oxleas NHS Foundation Trust Prescribing Guidelines* (9th edn) Informa Healthcare (pp. 505–507)

Core information

General principles
- Consider
  - Risk of relapse or deterioration in symptoms, severity of previous episodes
  - That stopping drug after pregnancy is confirmed may not remove risk of malformations
  - Risks of stopping a drug abruptly
  - Size of any increased risk
  - Risk in overdose

When prescribing
- Choose drugs with lower risk profiles, start at lowest effective dose and slowly increase
- Use monotherapy where possible

As alternatives use CBT/ interpersonal therapy (IPT) or an antipsychotic (preferably a low dose typical such as haloperidol, chlorpromazine or trifluoperazine)

For severe sleep problems try low dose chlorpromazine or amitryptiline

Do not forget ECT as an option

For rapid tranquilisation use short half life drugs, do not seclude after and modify restraint

Antipsychotics
- Raised prolactin reduces fertility with risperidone, amisulpride and sulpiride
- Gestational diabetes and weight gain with olanzapine
- Agranulocytosis with clozapine (theoretically)
- EPSEs with depot medication

Lithium
- Foetal heart defects (risk increases from 8 in 1000 to 60 in 1000, risk is in first trimester)
- Ebstein's anomaly (risk increases from 1 in 20,000 to 10 in 20,000, risk is in first trimester)
- Lithium readily enters breast milk to give high levels
- If lithium is continued, keep serum levels low and monitor closely

Antidepressants
- Lowest risks with amitryptiline, nortryptiline and Imipramine (but worse in overdose)
- Fluoxetine is best SSRI
- Foetal heart defects with paroxetine (risk in first trimester)
- Imipramine, nortryptiline and sertraline pass into breast milk less readily than citalopram and fluoxetine

Benzodiazepines
- Risk of cleft palate and other malformations
- Floppy baby syndrome in the neonate

Carbamazepine and lamotrigine
- Neural tube defects with Carbamazepine (risk increases from 6 in 10,000 to 20–50 in 10,000)
- Oral cleft risk (9 in 1000) with lamotrigine and dermatological problems if breastfeeding

Valproate
- Neural tube defect (spina bifida and anencephaly risk increases from 6 in 10,000 to 100–200 in 10,000)

If a foetus has been put at risk
- Confirm pregnancy, offer screening and counselling about pregnancy continuation and additional monitoring.
- Full paediatric assessment of the newborn and close monitoring during first few weeks after delivery
- Floppy baby syndrome, irritability, constant crying, shivering, restlessness, tremor, increased tone, feeding or sleeping problems and rarely seizures

If in doubt
  Seek advice from hospital pharmacy
  Avoid valproate in pregnancy if possible

Essential guidelines (Maudsley guidelines 2007)

During pregnancy
  Always discuss possibility of pregnancy with women of child-bearing potential
  Avoid drugs contraindicated in pregnancy especially valproate and carbamazepine
  Always take into consideration the risk of relapse when considering discontinuing
  psychotropic medication
  Try to avoid all drugs in the first trimester
  Ensure adequate foetal screening
Whilst breast-feeding
  Weigh the benefits of breast-feeding to the mother and infant against the risk of drug
  exposure in the infant
  Infants should be monitored for any specific adverse effects of the drugs as well as for
  feeding patterns and growth and development
  It is usually inappropriate to withhold treatment to allow breast-feeding Treatment of
  maternal illness is the highest priority
  Time the feeds to avoid peak drug levels in the milk or express milk to give later

REFERENCES

Gelder, M., Harrison, P. & Cowen, P. (2001) *Shorter Oxford Textbook of Psychiatry* (5th edn) Oxford University Press
    p. 523
Johnstone, E.C. & Cunningham Owens, D.G. et al. (eds) (2004) *Companion to Psychiatric Studies* (7th edn) Churchill
    Livingstone pp. 291–306 & 749–751
Joint Formulary Committee. British National Formulary (56th edn) British Medical Association and Royal
    Pharmaceutical Society of Great Britain pp. 802–837
King, D.J. (ed) (2004) *College Seminars Series: Seminars in Clinical Psychopharmacology* (2nd edn) The Royal College
    of Psychiatrists pp. 601–623
NICE Clinical Guidelines: Antenatal and postnatal mental health (2004) National Institute for Clinical Excellence
Taylor, D., Paton, C. & Kerwin, R. (2007) *The South London and Maudsley NHS Foundation Trust & Oxleas NHS
    Foundation Trust Prescribing Guidelines* (9th edn) Informa Healthcare pp. 365–387

ELECTRO-CONVULSIVE THERAPY (ECT)

Information giving

What it is

'ECT stands for electro-convulsive therapy.'

'It is a physical treatment which is mainly used for severe depression.'

'Because ECT therapy works by causing a seizure, it is performed under general anaesthetic. Medication is also given to relax your muscles.'

'During ECT a small safe pulse of modified electricity is passed through your brain. This is what produces the controlled seizure which lasts for a matter of seconds.'

'Often the only proof that the seizure has taken place is by looking at the EEG which is a tracing of your brain's activity.'

What it is not

'In the past large doses of electricity were given and anaesthesia was not as good. Some people also have memories of seeing ECT in films where the characters were awake during their treatment: this is far from today's reality.'

How does it work?

'ECT works by normalising levels of chemical messengers.'

Why is it better than medication?

'Research has shown that ECT can work even when antidepressants have failed. It also works faster, especially in more severe depressions.'

Risks

'The risks involved in having ECT are the same as having a minor procedure under a general anaesthetic. Serious problems occur in less than one in 50,000 treatments. The risks will be minimised by performing a physical examination and relevant tests such as blood tests and an ECG beforehand.'

Side effects

'Side effects of ECT are usually mild and short lasting. They include muscle pains, nausea, headache and feeling confused for a couple of hours.'

'Sometimes people experience some memory loss. This is mostly short-lived although there is some evidence that ECT may cause long-lasting memory impairment.'

How to minimise side effects

'When we give ECT we always start with the lowest dose and work upwards until the required clinical effect is seen. This is because different people need different doses. Taking this approach reduces the risk of side-effects.'

'During ECT two electrodes are usually placed on either side of the head. However if memory loss is a problem we sometimes place both electrodes on the same side of the head as this is thought to reduce memory loss.'

What will happen during ECT?

Before ECT

'Before you receive ECT you will be seen by an anaesthetist who will ask you some questions to make the process as safe as possible.'

'You will need to fast overnight as with any anaesthetic.'

'On the day you be taken to the ECT suite by one of the nurses where your psychiatrist and your anaesthetist will be waiting for you.'

During ECT

'You will be asked to lie on a couch and you will be given some oxygen. You will then be connected to some monitors which record things such as your blood pressure and your heart rate.'

'The anaesthetist will then give you some drugs through a drip. These include a muscle relaxant and the anaesthetic.'

'Once you are asleep, the ECT electrodes are attached and you will be given a dose. The seizure will last for less than one minute. Because your muscles will be relaxed the seizure will look more like a twitch.'

After ECT

'You will come around from the anaesthetic after a few moments. As you will feel drowsy, nursing staff will stay with you until you are ready to go back to the ward.'

How many sessions?

No fixed number, depends upon response, six to eight usually

Consent

'You will need to sign a consent form before you receive ECT. You may wish to discuss the treatment with family and friends before going ahead and you may change your mind at any time.'

'As ECT is very effective, it is sometimes the only option when people become very unwell, and therefore patient consent is not always possible. In such situations, it has to be given under The Mental Health Act and a second opinion doctor may need to be called in.'

Essential guidelines (NICE guidelines on ECT 2003)

Should only be used for

Severe and life threatening depression

Catatonia

Prolonged or severe mania

Patient should be assessed after each session

ECT should be stopped when response is achieved

REFERENCES

Gelder, M., Harrison, P. & Cowen, P. (2001) *Shorter Oxford Textbook of Psychiatry* (5th edn) (2001) Oxford University Press pp. 565–572

Johnstone, E.C. & Cunningham Owens, D.G. et al. (eds) (2004) *Companion to Psychiatric Studies* (7th edn) Churchill Livingstone pp. 439 & 647

King, D.J. (ed) (2004) *College Seminars Series: Seminars in Clinical Psychopharmacology* (2nd edn) The Royal College of Psychiatrists pp. 278–315

NICE *Clinical Guidelines: The clinical effectiveness and cost effectiveness of electroconvulsive Therapy (ECT) for depressive illness, schizophrenia, catatonia and mania.* (2003) National Institute for Clinical Excellence

Scott, A. (ed) *The ECT Handbook: The Third Report of the Royal College of Psychiatrists' Special Committee on ECT* (2nd edn) Gaskell

THE DEMENTIAS

Core diagnostic criteria (ICD-10)

Decline in memory most evident in the learning of new information, and decline in other cognitive abilities characterised by deterioration in judgement and thinking, such as planning and organizing, and in the general processing of information.

Awareness of the environment (i.e. absence of clouding of consciousness).

Decline in emotional control or motivation, or a change in social behaviour manifest as at least one of the following: emotional lability, irritability, apathy and coarsening of social behaviour.

Core information

Investigations

Blood tests (including full blood count, erythrocyte sedimentation rate, urea, creatinine, electrolytes, liver function tests, thyroid function tests, Vitamin B_{12} and folate)

Blood glucose

Cholesterol

Syphilis serology

Mid-stream urinalysis (MSU)

Electrocardiogram (ECG) and echocardiogram

Chest x-ray

Electroencephalogram (EEG)

Neuroimaging e.g. CT, MRI and SPET scan

Key phrases

Clinical description

'Dementia is the most usual cause of memory problems in later life. It mainly affects older people.'

'As well as memory difficulties, dementia can also lead to word-finding difficulties, difficulties with skills such as dressing and using cutlery, failure of intelligence, judgement and logic, personality changes such as becoming withdrawn and suspicious, anxiety and depression, wandering behaviour and becoming dependent on others for care.'

'There are several causes of dementia, but the commonest is Alzheimer's disease. The next commonest cause is vascular dementia, although people may have a mix of both. The other causes of dementia are far less common.'

Alzheimer's disease

Description

'In Alzheimer's disease, brain cells are lost and are replaced by abnormal deposits, leading to a worsening of normal brain functioning.'

Diagnosis

'Alzheimer's disease should only be diagnosed in people whose dementia has come on slowly. Before a diagnosis can be made, doctors must exclude other causes of dementia such as vitamin deficiencies, thyroid problems and neurological disease.'

Prognosis

'Unfortunately, Alzheimer's disease always gets steadily worse.'

'The forgetfulness becomes more problematic, and eventually people with this sort of dementia may even get lost in familiar surroundings.'

'As the disease progresses, people may fail to recognise their loved ones.'

'The illness usually runs a course of between five and ten years, but this does vary.'

Risk of developing Alzheimer's disease

'We are probably all at risk of developing Alzheimer's disease if we live long enough.'

'The risk of developing Alzheimer's disease increases with age.'

'Studies show that first degree relatives of someone with Alzheimer's disease who developed the disorder at any time up to the age of 85, are about three to four times more likely to develop the disease than other people.'

'There is a familial form of Alzheimer's disease in which 50% of each generation gets the disease by their early mid-life, but cases of this are rare.'

Genetic testing

'Early onset dementia can be genetic. If families have three or more members affected before the age of 60 years, then they might benefit from seeing a genetic specialist. In the case of familial Alzheimer's disease, a DNA diagnosis may be made in seven out of ten families.'

Management

Drugs to enhance memory (acetylcholinesterase inhibitors)

See *Drug treatments for dementia* sheet

Antipsychotics

Modest effect on difficult behaviours in dementia

However antipsychotics may increase the risk of stroke, precipitate an irreversible syndrome of Parkinsonism and hasten cognitive decline when given to individuals with dementia.

Therefore antipsychotics should only be used if the behavioural problems are severe.

Antidepressants

SSRIs and preferred for treating depression in dementia and they may also help with agitation. Other antidepressants may be used but tricyclic antidepressants are best avoided.

Ginkgo biloba

Research shows that whilst Gingko biloba may improve memory and concentration in individuals who have dementia, the effects are minimal.

Vascular dementia

Description

'In vascular dementia there is damage to the brain's circulation, leading to a worsening of normal brain functioning.'

Diagnosis

'People who are diagnosed with vascular dementia usually have evidence of neurological disease.'

'The main example of such disease is stroke.'

'Physical symptoms and signs, which make a diagnosis of vascular dementia possible, include a one-sided weakness of the limbs, changes in muscle reflexes or nerve palsy.'

Prognosis

'People with vascular dementia usually deteriorate in a stepwise fashion. This means that whilst every now and then their function seems to deteriorate quickly, in between these times they may remain stable for some time.'

'This pattern is different to the pattern seen in Alzheimer's disease where affected individuals deteriorate steadily without these periods of stability.'

Risk of developing vascular dementia

'It is impossible to predict who will get vascular dementia and who will not. Apart from some very rare genetic forms of vascular dementia (e.g. CADASIL) there is little evidence that it runs in families.'

Management
  Antidepressants
    Antidepressants should be considered for associated depression
  Control vascular risk factors
    Antihypertensive medication
    Statins
    Anticoagulant medication
    Liaise with medical specialist e.g. care of elderly physician
  Health promotion
    Advise to stop smoking/drinking alcohol

Dementia in Parkinson's disease and Lewy body dementia

Description
  'Dementia in Parkinson's disease and Lewy body dementia are probably best thought of as an overlap between Alzheimer's disease and Parkinson's disease. With both of these conditions, brain cells are lost and are replaced by abnormal deposits, leading to a worsening of normal brain functioning.'

Diagnosis
  'The diagnosis is clinical. People who have dementia in Parkinson's disease and Lewy body dementia often have different sorts of symptoms from people with other forms of dementia like Alzheimer's disease. Examples of such symptoms include visual hallucinations—which is when people see things that aren't really there—rigid joints, slowness of movement and tremor—the symptoms which are seen in Parkinson's disease. People's ability to think clearly and function properly may fluctuate dramatically, and they can also be prone to drowsiness and falls.'

Prognosis
  'Whilst many patients may respond well to medications in the short term, the condition will inevitably progress over time. The outlook for dementia in Parkinson's disease and Lewy body dementia is generally poor, as there is no specific treatment to reverse the progression of disease.'

Management
  Drugs to enhance memory (acetylcholinesterase inhibitors)
    See *Drug Treatments for Dementia*
  Antipsychotics
    Whilst antipsychotics might usually be considered for controlling the agitation seen in dementia, there is a risk of neuroleptic sensitivity with even atypical antipsychotics and they are usually best avoided.
  Antidepressants
    SSRIs are preferred when treating depression in dementia in Parkinson's disease and Lewy body dementia.

Frontotemporal dementia and Pick's disease

Description
  'Frontotemporal dementia and Pick's disease are types of dementia which mainly affect the front region of the brain. They are thought to be caused by a loss of brain cells and an abnormal build up of chemical deposits in the brain.'

Diagnosis
  'At the beginning, the symptoms may be very general and so it is not always easy to pick the diagnosis up. And as with other dementias, it is important to exclude underlying physical illness. Brain scans may be used to look for the particular patterns seen in these types of

dementia. However, the most helpful information is often the clinical picture. Symptoms which suggest a diagnosis of frontotemporal dementia or Pick's disease include, amongst many, changes in behaviour and personality, lack of inhibition and impairment of speech.'

Prognosis

'Whilst the deterioration seen in frontotemporal dementia and Pick's disease may be slow, unfortunately the condition always gets steadily worse. Medication and therapies may be helpful but there is no specific treatment and they do not prevent the inevitable disease progression.'

Risk of developing frontotemporal dementia

'Research shows that in about half of all cases frontotemporal dementia there is a family history. First-degree relatives are estimated to be three to four times more likely to develop frontotemporal dementia before the age of 80 than healthy controls.'

Management

Antipsychotics

Antidepressants

Social support and nursing care (for all dementias)

'Help is available from both social services and the health service. For example, people are offered the chance to attend day services where they can share a meal with others or where they might join reminiscence groups.'

'Home support is also available, which may be arranged to help with tasks such as dressing and washing.'

'It is also possible to arrange short stays in a residential home to give both the individual and their carer a break.'

'Further down the road, it is sometimes necessary to look for a permanent residential placement.'

Support groups

Alzheimer's Society (also has information regarding other dementias)

Help the Aged

Age Concern

Essential guidelines (NICE guidelines on dementia 2006)

People with mild to moderate dementia should be offered participation in structured group cognitive stimulation programmes.

For challenging behaviour in dementia, if there is severe distress or risk of harm to self or others, then antipsychotics may be considered.

REFERENCES

Butler, R. & Pitt, B. (ed) (1998) *College Seminars Series: Seminars in Old Age Psychiatry* Royal College of Psychiatrists (pp. 49–77)

Cooper, J. (ed) (2004) *Pocket Guide to the ICD-10: Classification of Mental and Behavioural Disorders.* Churchill Livingstone pp. 28–44

Gelder, M., Harrison, P. & Cowen, P. *Shorter Oxford Textbook of Psychiatry* (5th edn) Oxford University Press pp. 498–511

Jacoby, R. & Oppenheimer, C. (ed) (2002) *Psychiatry in the Elderly* (3rd edn) Oxford University Press pp. 509–543

Liddell, M.B., Lovestone, S. & Owen, M.J.(2001) *Genetic risk of Alzheimer's disease: advising relatives* British Journal of Psychiatry, **178**, 7–11

NICE Clinical Guidelines: Dementia.(2006) National Institute for Clinical Excellence

Stevens, M., van Duijn, C.M., Kamphorst, W. et al. (1998) *Familial aggregation in frontotemporal dementia* Neurology, **50**(6), 1541–1545

Information giving

Description

'There are two groups of drugs used to help combat the early signs of dementia. The drugs which make up the first group are called acetylcholinesterase inhibitors. The drugs belonging to this group are Donepezil, Galantamine and Rivastigmine. There is only one drug which belongs to the other group and it is called Memantine. At present it is not recommended for use in the NHS.'

'Acetylcholinesterase inhibitors do not cure dementia, but they are thought to improve certain symptoms.'

Indications

'Acetylcholinesterase inhibitors, are given to people with moderate dementia. All three have similar clinical effects. They improve memory, attention and motivation although they have only been shown to have a modest effect.'

Contraindications

'Some people who have stomach ulcers or problems with their heart such as heart block will not be able to have this medication.'

Mode of action

'Acetylcholinesterase inhibitors work by reducing the breakdown of acetylcholine. Acetylcholine is a chemical in the brain. This chemical is reduced in people with Alzheimer's disease and other related dementias. So by boosting the levels of acetylcholine, acetylcholinesterase inhibitors boost memory. Unfortunately acetylcholinesterase only help the symptoms, they have not been shown to delay the progress of the disease.'

Side effects

'Acetylcholinesterase inhibitors are usually well tolerated but they can sometimes cause nausea, vomiting, reduced appetite, diarrhoea, tiredness, poor sleep and headache.'

Dose

Donepezil (Aricept) initially 5mg once daily at bedtime, increased if necessary after one month to 10mg daily

Galantamine (Reminyl) initially 4mg twice daily for four weeks increased to 8mg twice daily for four weeks; maintenance 8–12mg twice daily

Rivastigmine (Exelon) initially 1.5mg twice daily, increased in steps of 1.5mg twice daily according to response/tolerance; usual range 3–6mg twice daily

Preparations

All three medications are available in either a tablet or capsule form

Galantamine and Rivastigmine are also available in an oral solution

Galantamine is also available in a modified release formulation (Reminyl XL)

Time course

'The length of time each person takes these medications differs from person to person.'

'It is unclear how long people continue to benefit from them.'

'However, generally speaking, they are usually effective for 9–12 months and sometimes for several years.'

The evidence base

'Studies have shown that the effect of acetylcholinesterase inhibitors is small to moderate.'

Essential guidelines (NICE guidelines on anti-dementia drugs amended 2007)

The drug should only be continued while the patient's MMSE score remains at or above ten points (and below 20) and their global, functional and behavioural condition remains at a level where the drug is considered to be having a worthwhile effect.

Patient should be reviewed every six months and carer's views should be sought. Acetylcholinesterase inhibitors may still be considered for patients who score more than 20 on the MMSE if their functional ability or social function is significantly impaired. Acetylcholinesterase inhibitors may still be considered for patients who score less than ten on the MMSE if the score may be explained by factors such as low premorbid attainment or linguistic difficulties.

REFERENCES

Jacoby, R. & Oppenheimer, C. (ed) (2002) *Psychiatry in the Elderly* (3rd edn) Oxford University Press pp. 509–532

Joint Formulary Committee. British National Formulary (56th edn) (2008) British Medical Association and Royal Pharmaceutical Society of Great Britain

NICE Clinical Guidelines: Dementia (2006) National Institute for Clinical Excellence

Rockwood, K. *Size of the treatment effect on cognition of cholinesterase inhibition in Alzheimer's disease* (2004) Journal of Neurology, Neurosurgery and Psychiatry, **75**, 677–685

DELIRIUM

Core diagnostic criteria (ICD-10)

Impairment of consciousness and attention.

Impairment of immediate recall and recent memory with relative intact remote memory, as well as disorientation in time, place or person.

Psychomotor disturbance: unpredictable shifts from hypoactivity to hyperactivity, increased reaction time, increased or decreased flow of speech, or enhanced startle reaction.

Disturbance of sleep or of the sleep-wake cycle: insomnia, nocturnal worsening of symptoms, disturbing dreams and nightmares which may continue as hallucinations or illusions after awakening.

Symptoms have a rapid onset and fluctuate over the course of the day.

Information giving

Clinical description

'Delirium is a sudden, fluctuating, and usually reversible disturbance of mental function.'

'It is characterised by changes in consciousness.'

'It is different from dementia, although people with dementia may also become delirious.'

Causes

'Whilst delirium is not just a disorder of older people, old age, frailty and an existing diagnosis of dementia make someone more likely to become delirious.'

'There are numerous causes of delirium. They include medication, alcohol, infection, head injury and constipation.'

Diagnosis

'There is no test for delirium, although certain tests may be useful in determining the cause. The diagnosis is entirely clinical.'

Prognosis

'Many cases of delirium recover rapidly but there is a 25% mortality rate at three months.'

'There is no evidence that delirium progresses to dementia.'

Management

'Delirium is a medical emergency and it is important to identify and treat the underlying cause.'

'Steps are taken to relieve distress and agitation and to prevent exhaustion. For example, efforts are made to reorientate the patient. For this reason we try to limit the number of staff working with the patient and try to avoid unnecessary changes in staff during a nursing shift. People with delirium are often nursed in a separate room and relatives are encouraged to visit regularly to reassure the patient. Simple things such as appropriate lighting and being able to see a clock are also important.'

'People with delirium may need medication to treat the underlying cause, but sometimes they might also need medication to control their distress and to enable them to sleep. When medication is needed it is introduced carefully so that no more than the minimum effective dose is given.'

Essential guidelines

The National Institute for Clinical Excellence (NICE) is currently drafting *The diagnosis, prevention and management of delirium*, which is due to be published during April 2010.

REFERENCES

Cooper, J. (ed) (2004) *Pocket Guide to the ICD-10: Classification of Mental and Behavioural Disorders* Churchill Livingstone pp. 46–48

Gelder, M., Harrison, P. & Cowen, P. (2001) *Shorter Oxford Textbook of Psychiatry* (5th edn) Oxford University Press
   pp. 329–330
Jacoby, R. & Oppenheimer, C. (ed) (2002) *Psychiatry in the Elderly* (3rd edn) Oxford University Press
   pp. 592–615
NICE Clinical Guidelines: Dementia (2006) National Institute for Clinical Excellence

3.3 LEARNING DISABILITY (LD)

LEARNING DISABILITY AND MENTAL HEALTH

Learning disability

Core information

IQ and severity of learning disability (LD)
Mild = 50–69
Moderate = 35–49
Severe = 20–34
Profound = <20

A diagnosis of mental retardation within ICD-10 (F70–F79) may be made by learning disability psychiatrists but ideally would be confirmed by formal psychometric testing by a clinical psychologist with learning disability experience.

Assessing psychiatric morbidity in learning disability
Instruments
e.g. Psychiatric Assessment Schedule for Adults with Developmental Disorder (PAS-ADD)

The Mental Health Act (MHA), The Mental Capacity Act (MCA) and 'The Bournewood Gap'

Core information

The Mental Health Act 1983 recognised four distinct categories of mental disorder:
Mental illness
Mental impairment
Severe mental impairment
Psychopathic disorder

To satisfy the criteria for detention for treatment it was necessary, with the latter three categories, to also have evidence of an association with abnormally aggressive or seriously irresponsible conduct. In the Mental Health Act 2007 this has been retained for learning disability only.

The Bournewood case concerned a 49-year-old man with autism who was a patient at Bournewood Hospital in 1997. He was not detained under the Mental Health Act but informally and under common law 'best interests'. The European Court of Human Rights held that he had been held unlawfully.

'The Bournewood Gap' is a phrase used to describe this grey area in the law when someone without capacity was neither actively attempting to leave the hospital nor consenting to being there.

The Mental Health Act 2007 aimed to address this problem and introduced procedures for 'Deprivations of Liberty' safeguards (DoLs). These procedures are lengthy and complex. The Mental Health Act 2007 also introduced changes to guardianship so that there is now a 'take and convey' option to return people to the place where it has been decided they should reside. With this option the criteria for detention must be met.

REFERENCES

Fraser, W. & Kerr, M. (eds) (2003) *College Seminars Series: Seminars in The Psychiatry of Learning Disability* Royal College of Psychiatrists pp. 307–318

The Mental Health Act 2007

The Mental Capacity Act 2005.

Core information

Down's syndrome in the ICD-10 = Q90

First described by John Langdon Down in 1866

May be due to

    Trisomy 21 (95% of cases)

    Mosaicism (responsible for 1–2% of cases)

    Translocation (2–3% of cases)

Epidemiology of Down's syndrome

    Incidence = 1 per 800 to 1 per 1000

    Effect of maternal age on incidence

        20–24yrs = 1/1500

        35–39 = 1/200

        >45 = 1/19

The learning disability

    Affected persons most commonly have mild to moderate LD

    A smaller number have a severe to profound LD

Prognosis

    Life expectancy around 50 years

Physical health problems

    Cardiac abnormalities e.g. septal defects

    Impaired hearing

    Hypothyroidism

Alzheimer's disease in Down's syndrome prevalence

    30–39 yrs = 2–3%

    40–49 yrs = 9–10%

    50–59 yrs = 36–40%

    60–69 yrs = 55%

Assessment

    The diagnosis of dementia in people with LD is difficult (especially in early stages) because of the lack of reliable and standardised criteria and diagnostic procedures.

Examples of dementia screening tools

    Dementia Screening Questionnaire for Individuals with Intellectual Disabilities (DSQIID)

    Dementia Scale for Down Syndrome (DSDS)

    Dementia Questionnaire for People with Learning Disabilities(DLD)

    MMSE is of limited use

REFERENCES

Fraser, W. & Kerr, M. (eds). (2003) *College Seminars Series: Seminars in The Psychiatry of Learning Disability*. Royal College of Psychiatrists pp. 267–286

Prasher, V.P. (1994) *Age specific prevalence, thyroid dysfunction and depressive symptomology in adult's with Down's syndrome and dementia*. International Journal of Geriatic Psychiatry. **10**, 25–31

Holland, A.J. et al. (1998) *Population based study of the prevalence and presentation of dementia in adults with Down's syndrome*. British Journal of Psychiatry. **172**, 493–498

CHALLENGING BEHAVIOUR

Core information

Causes of agitation in a person with LD
- Environmental causes
    - Too hot/cold
    - Wet
    - Tired
    - Hungry/thirsty
- Situational causes
    - Frightened
    - Over-stimulated
    - Under-stimulated/bored
    - Lonely/wanting attention
    - Frustration due to difficulty communicating needs/wants
- Visual impairment
- Hearing impairment
- Side effects of medication
    - Sedation
    - Extra pyramidal side effects (EPSEs)
- Pain/discomfort
    - E.g. osteoarthritis is common in Down's Syndrome
- Psychiatric causes
    - Depression
    - Pseudodementia
    - Adjustment disorder
    - Bereavement reaction
    - Anxiety disorder
    - Psychosis
- Other dementia
    - Lewy Body Dementia
    - Reversible dementia due to B_{12} or folate deficiency
- Endocrine causes
    - Hypothyroidism
    - Hyperthyroidism

Management of challenging behaviour
- Observation
- Consider use of ABC charts (Antecedent→Behaviour→Consequence)

REFERENCES

Fraser, W. & Kerr, M. (eds). (2003) *College Seminars Series: Seminars in The Psychiatry of Learning Disability.* Royal College of Psychiatrists pp. 155–169

LEARNING DISABILITY AND OFFENDING

Core information

Issues to be considered

Does the subject have a LD and to what degree?

Is the subject's behaviour intrinsically linked to his LD?

Does the behaviour fall within the category of 'abnormally aggressive or seriously irresponsible conduct'?

Is the person suggestible?

Is there a mental disorder in addition?

Does this warrant detention in its own right?

Is the subject fit to plead?

Was an appropriate adult present during police interview?

In the case of homicide, is diminished responsibility an issue?

Certain offences such as arson and sexual offending are overrepresented in the learning disability population.

Information giving

Management options for the learning disabled offender

Treatment in the community is the mainstay of recommended disposals for people with LD.

The statutory options are

Probation order with a condition of treatment

Supervision order under the Criminal Procedures Insanity Act (CPIA) 1991

Guardianship under Section 37 or 7 of MHA 1983

Regardless of the statutory option, the treatment is likely to include

Residential placement with family or in statutory, voluntary or independent sector

Educational provision

Structured day activities (reduces boredom and tendency to re-offend)

Therapeutic intervention by NHS, social services and/or probation service e.g. sexual counselling, CBT, group psychotherapy (to address denial, minimization, responsibility and victim awareness), and antilibidinals.

Monitoring of mental state (to treat mental illness if coexistent e.g. antipsychotics)

The Sexual Offender Treatment Programme unsuitable for IQ <80.

Coordination and supervision of the overall package of care

Treatment may also be provided in the prison service or under Section 37 MHA 1983 at local facilities, medium secure units and special hospitals (Rampton has an LD service).

REFERENCES

Fraser, W. & Kerr, M. (ed) (2003) *College Seminars Series: Seminars in The Psychiatry of Learning Disability*. Royal College of Psychiatrists pp. 287–306

Stone, J.H., Roberts, M., O'Grady, J., Taylor, A.V. (eds) (2000) *Faulk's Basic Forensic Psychiatry* (3rd edn) Blackwell Publishing

Chiswick, D. & Cope, R. (eds).(1998) *College Seminars Series: Seminars in Practical Forensic Psychiatry*. The Royal College of Psychiatrists pp. 71–75

EPILEPSY AND LEARNING DISABILITY

Key phrases

'When did you first notice something was wrong?'
'What happened?'
'Did they lose consciousness?'
'Were there any unusual or jerky movements?'
'How long did this go on for?'
'Can you think what may have triggered this off?'
'Were there any warning signs?'
'How often does this happen?'
'Does anything like this happen to anyone else in the family?'

Information giving

'About 20 per cent of people with a learning disability have a history of epilepsy, compared with about five per cent in the general population. The rate of epilepsy increases as the severity of the learning disability increases.'
'It can sometimes be more difficult to treat in people with a learning disability.'

Core information

Types of seizures :
Primary generalised seizures [affects both sides (whole of) of the brain from onset]
    Absence seizures (petit mal)
        Simple absence seizures with episodes of staring that usually last only a few seconds
        Complex absence seizures which also involve some motor activity, commonly blinking, finger rubbing and mouth movements
    Myoclonic seizures
        Brief shock-like jerks of a muscle or group of muscles. Usually involves the neck, shoulders, arms or face.
    Atonic seizures (drop attacks)
        Sudden loss of muscle tone. Usually results in a fall but with consciousness remaining.
    Tonic seizures
        Sudden stiffening of muscle groups, often causing falls but retaining consciousness.
    Clonic seizures
        Rhythmic jerking movements of the arms and legs (contraction then relaxation of muscle groups).
    Tonic clonic seizures (grand mal)
        Stiffening followed by rhythmic jerking movements.
Partial seizures (in one area of the brain only)
    Simple partial seizures
    These vary widely from person to person but consciousness remains and there is memory for the event.
        Motor seizures - can get isolated jerking or stiffening that may spread or can get coordinated actions such as laughing or hand movements.
        Sensory seizures - changes in any of the senses e.g. can smell, taste, hear, feel or see things that are not there (hallucinations) or have illusions.
        Autonomic seizures - can include changes in heart rate, sweating, unpleasant or strange stomach sensations.

Psychic seizures - can change how people think, feel or experience, can include déja vu (a feeling that something has happened before) or jamais vu (a feeling that something is new when it isn't)

Complex partial seizures

Also focal but with loss of awareness and typically occur in temporal lobe area. Can include complex actions such as walking into traffic or removing clothes.

Secondary generalised seizures

Begin as a partial seizure and become generalised usually resulting in a tonic clonic seizure.

Essential guidelines (NICE guidelines on '*The epilepsies: diagnosis and management of the epilepsies in adults in primary and secondary care*' October 2004)

All adults with a recent-onset suspected seizure should be seen urgently by a specialist to ensure precise and early diagnosis and initiation of therapy as appropriate to their needs. Seizure type(s) and epilepsy syndrome, aetiology and co-morbidity should be determined. The AED (anti-epileptic drug) treatment strategy should be individualised according to the seizure type, epilepsy syndrome, co-medication and co-morbidity, the individual's lifestyle, and the preferences of the individual, and their family and/or carers as appropriate. All individuals with epilepsy should have a regular structured review.

REFERENCES

Gelder, M. Harrison, P. & Cowen, P. (2001) *Shorter Oxford Textbook of Psychiatry* (5th edn) Oxford University Press pp. 346–350

Fraser, W. & Kerr, M. (eds).(2003) *College Seminars Series: Seminars in The Psychiatry of learning Disability*. Royal College of Psychiatrists pp. 239–249

Epilepsy.com http://www.epilepsy.com/epilepsy/types_seizures (Accessed 4 December 2008)

NICE Clinical Guidelines (2004) *The epilepsies: diagnosis and management of the epilepsies in adults in primary and secondary care*. National Institute for Clinical Excellence

AUTISTIC SPECTRUM DISORDER

Key phrases

'What difficulties does he have that you have noticed?'
    Started before age of three
        'When were you first concerned there may be something wrong with your child?'
Major difficulties
    'Does he have difficulty expressing himself or understanding others?'
    'Does he find it difficult interacting with others?'
    'Can he use his imagination to play?'
Social interaction
    'Is there anything unusual about his eye contact?'
    'Can he read facial expressions and social situations?'
    'Does he use body posture or gestures?'
    'Does he have friends?'
    'How does he respond to the emotions of others?'
    'Does he share experiences with others?'
Communication
    'Does he speak?' if not 'Does he make up for this with gestures or mime?'
    'Is he interested in communicating with others?'
    'Is he repetitive in his speech?'
    'Does he pretend or use "make believe"?'
Stereotyped, repetitive behaviour
    'Is there anything he is particularly interested in?'
    'Is there anything he is very particular about?'
    'Are there any routines or rituals he has to follow?'
    'Does he make any unusual movements such as spinning, rocking or hand flapping?'
    'Does he use toys in an unusual way, such as taking them apart?'
Asperger's syndrome
    No general delay or retardation in language or in cognitive development
    'Is he very clumsy?'
General
    'How are you coping with all of this?'
    'How are your other children?'
    'Does he have any medical problems?'

Information giving

'It seems as though your child may be on the autistic spectrum.'
'We think of autism as being a spectrum and children are affected to varying degrees. We need to spend more time with him to discover more about how exactly he is affected.'
Co-morbidity
    Learning disability (80%), Epilepsy (30%), Hearing impairment (20%)
    What else could it be?
        Rett's syndrome (if female), social anxiety, severe neglect
Management
    Social
        Teach to follow routines, to develop communication abilities
        Assistance and support for parents, practical advice, respite
        National Autistic Society for post diagnosis information and support

Behavioural

    Functional Analysis (Antecedent → Behaviour → Consequence)

    Teach to tolerate adult guidance and intrusion

Educational

    Structured educational programme, appropriate schooling

Pharmacology

    No medication has proven efficacy

    Risperidone for hyperactivity, impulsivity and aggression or SSRIs

REFERENCES

Gowers, S. (ed). (2005) *College Seminars Series: Seminars in Child and Adolescent Psychiatry* (2nd edn) Royal College of Psychiatrists pp. 124–144

Goodman, R. & Scott, S. *Child Psychiatry* (2nd edn) (2005) Blackwell pp. 43–51

Cooper, J. (ed.). (2004) *Pocket Guide to the ICD-10: Classification of Mental and Behavioural Disorders* Churchill Livingstone. pp. 262–288

HYPERKINETIC DISORDER

Core diagnostic criteria (ICD-10)

Need symptoms in all three areas of inattention, hyperactivity and impulsivity

Core diagnostic criteria (DSM-IV)

Can be mainly inattention symptoms to be ADHD
If symptoms in all three areas is severe ADHD

Key phrases

'What difficulties does he have that you have noticed?'
Inattention
    'Does he tend to ignore details or make careless errors?'
    'Can he sustain attention in tasks or play?'
    'Do you ever feel he is not listening?'
    'Does he ever fail to complete instructions?'
    'Do you feel he is poor at organizing?'
    'Does he avoid tasks that require sustained mental effort such as housework?'
    'Does he often lose things?'
    'Is he easily distracted?'
    'Is he forgetful?'
Hyperactivity (needs three)
    'Does he often fidget or squirm on his seat?'
    'Can he sit down with the family and complete a meal?'
    'Does he ever leave his seat when not supposed to?'
    'Does he often run or climb?' 'Do you feel this is ever inappropriate or excessive?'
    'Does he have difficulty playing quietly?'
    'Do you feel he is always on the go?'
Impulsivity (needs one)
    'Does he often blurt out answers to questions before the end of the question?'
    'Does he have difficulty waiting in line or waiting turn?'
    'Does he often interrupt or intrude in on others?'
    'Would you say he talks excessively?'
Pervasive across situations
    'Does he behave in this way in different situations?'
    'Would you say he is worse at home or at school?'
Persistent across time (six months)
    'How long has this been going on for?'
    'Have things gotten worse, better or stayed the same?'
No autism or affective disorder
    'Is he medically well?'
    'Has he ever been diagnosed with anything?'
    'How does he interact with other children?'
    'Have you noticed any language problems?'
    'How is his mood?'
    'How is his sleep?'
    'How is his appetite?'
Onset before age of seven
    'When did you first notice these difficulties?'

Effect on functioning
'Do these difficulties cause distress or prevent him from doing anything?'
'Does he get invited to play or to parties?'
Conduct disorder screen
'Does he get into trouble at school?'
'Is he ever aggressive?'
'Is he disobedient?'
Others
'How are other children in the family doing?'
'Does he ever put himself or others in danger?'

Information giving

How common
Affects about 1 in 20 worldwide (5%) aged under 19. 1 in 50 in the UK
60% estimated to retain symptoms into adulthood
Symptoms (as per previous section)
Three areas of inattention, impulsivity and hyperactivity
Different types and names depending on which symptoms are dominant
Aetiology
Probably not one cause
Genetics, environmental factors e.g. alcohol in utero and maternal smoking, also
premature birth
Role of food additives not clear
Some evidence that affects non-ADHD children causing hyperactivity symptoms
Investigations/assessment
Based on thorough history and social assessment. Home Hyperactivity Scale, Connor's
Teacher Rating Scale, Strength and Difficulty Questionnaire
Management through medication
Methylphenidate
Methylphenidate immediate release (Ritalin) – 5mg to 60mg
Methylphenidate controlled release (Concerta XL) – 18mg to 54mg
Methylphenidate CR, capsule which can be opened to extract liquid centre
(Equasym XL) – 10mg to 60mg
Methylphenidate is a stimulant, a controlled drug with abuse potential
Side effects: insomnia, mood and appetite changes, agitation, anxiety, psychosis, cardiac
effects, tics, possible effect on height but controversial (consider use of growth charts if
concerned), and lowering of seizure threshold.
Dexamphetamine
Stimulant, not often used
Atomoxetine
0.5mg/kg/day to 1.2mg/kg/day (<70kg),
40mg to 80mg (>70kg)
Side effects: most commonly reduced appetite, agitation, increased risk of self harm/
suicidality, dry mouth, nausea, vomiting, and constipation. Need to monitor liver function.
How long for?
Have regular 'medication holidays', if on a stimulant, to see if still needed, usually during
school holidays
Can continue into adulthood if required
Psychosocial
Behavioural techniques, lifestyle changes e.g. diet

Psychology
　　anxiety management, CBT (individual or group), family therapy, social skills training
Support groups
　　National Attention Deficit Disorder Information and Support Service (ADDISS)
What will the school do?
　　Made aware, given techniques and advice, extra support and time
What else could it be?
　　Epilepsy
　　Hearing problems
　　Reading difficulties
　　OCD
　　Tourette's
　　Autistic Spectrum Disorder
　　Poor sleep
Co-morbidity
　　Anxiety
　　Depression
　　Conduct disorder
　　Specific learning difficulty
Prognosis
　　Can live a full and normal life with help

Essential guidelines (NICE guidelines on hyperkinetic disorder 2006)

Can use methylphenidate, atomoxetine or dexamphetamine
Consider modified release
Decide on an individual basis based on
　　Preference of parent and young person
　　Comorbidity such as tics
　　Side effects
　　Compliance
　　Potential for drug diversion

REFERENCES

ADDISS.co.uk, ADHD information services. http://www.addiss.co.uk [Accessed 27 October 2008]

Goodman, R. & Scott, S. I, (2nd edn) (2005) Blackwell Publishing pp. 43–51

NICE Clinical Guidelines (2006) *Methylphenidate, atomoxetine and dexamfetamine for attention deficit hyperactivity disorder (ADHD) in children and adolescents.* National Institute for Clinical Excellence

Joint Formulary Committee. British National Formulary. (56th edn) (2008) British Medical Association and Royal Pharmaceutical Society of Great Britain pp. 211–213

Cooper, J. (ed) (2004). *Pocket Guide to the ICD-10: Classification of Mental and Behavioural Disorders.* Churchill Livingstone pp. 289–325

SCHOOL REFUSAL

School refusal is a presentation for a diverse range of diagnoses particularly anxiety disorders, ASD and mood disorders. Various family difficulties can also present with children 'school refusing'.

Key phrases

'When did this start?'
'How often is he refusing to go to school?'
'What reasons does he give?'
'What does he do when not at school?'
'Have they recently changed school?'
'Can you think of any triggers?'
'Any separation anxiety when younger?'
'Any physical complaints such as stomachache, headache, nausea?'
'Are there any stresses in the family at the moment?'
'Are you aware of any fallings out with friends or bullying?'
'Any difficulties with teachers?'
'How are you?'
Possible causes
   'Were there any problems with her birth or development?'
   'Does he ever appear anxious?'
   'Are there ever any panic attacks?'
   'How is her mood/sleep/appetite?'
   'Does he ever seem fixated on any one thing such as washing or checking?'
   'Does he have any phobias that you know of?'
   'Does he ever drink alcohol or take any illicit substances?'
Management
   Medical
      Treat underlying mental illness or disability
   Psychological
      Functional Analysis
      CBT
      Anxiety management
      Family therapy
   Educational
      Return to school as soon as possible
      Arrange educational support
   Social
      School liaison to provide reintegration package
      Address any communication difficulties
      Social and communication skills training
      Practical family support
      Empowerment training for performance anxiety
      If bullied then look at specific strategies e.g. assertiveness training, specific coping skills, peer refusal training
   Pharmacological
      Can consider use of fluoxetine to treat severe anxiety or depression. Sertraline or citalopram can be used second line.

Essential guidelines (NICE guidelines on depression in children 2005)

Treat for six months minimum

Mild depression

    Self help or CBT

Moderate or severe depression

    Fluoxetine 10–20mg in 12–18 year-olds and with caution in 5–11 year-olds

    Can also use sertraline or citalopram

Advise all to discontinue St John's Wort

REFERENCES

Gowers, S. (ed.). *College Seminars Series: Seminars in Child and Adolescent Psychiatry,* (2nd edn) (2005) Royal College of Psychiatrists pp. 158–173

Goodman, R. & Scott, S. *Child Psychiatry,* (2nd edn) (2005) Blackwell pp. 78–83

NICE Clinical Guidelines (2005) *Depression in children and young people.* National Institute for Clinical Excellence

ENCOPRESIS AND ENURESIS

Key phrases (encopresis)

'What difficulties does he have that you have noticed?'
'At what age did he first achieve continence of stool?'
'Is he ever incontinent of stool?'
'When did this start?'
'Where does this happen?'
'How often is this happening?'
'Is it a large amount?'
'Is the stool hard or soft?'
'Where is the stool deposited?'
'Do you think he is constipated?'
'Do you notice him holding in his stool?'
'Does he ever complain of abdominal pain?'
'What is his diet like?'
'Do you know of any physical problems?'
'Can you think of any reason why this might be happening?'
'Any recent stress in the family?'
'What have you done to try to prevent him behaving like this?'
'Have you had any professional help in the past?'

Key phrases (enuresis)

'What difficulties does he have that you have noticed?'
'At what age did he achieve continence of urine?'
'Is he ever incontinent of urine?'
'When did this start?'
'Is he wet by day or by night?'
'Where does this happen?'
'How often is this happening?'
'Do you know of any physical problems?'
'Has he ever been tested for a urinary tract infection?'
'Is there any history of epilepsy or seizures?'
'Can you think of any reason why this might be happening?'
'Any recent stress in the family?'
'What have you done to try to prevent him behaving like this?'
'Have you had any professional help in the past?'

Information giving

'No-one is to blame here.'
Rule out physical causes
    'Usually we like to rule out physical problems by doing a few tests. These could include bloods, abdominal X-ray, urine dipstick, height and weight measurement, abdominal palpation, looking for anal fissures, irritation or faecal impaction. We may also get advice from a paediatrician if thought necessary.'
Management
    Medical
        Fluid restriction in the afternoon or evening
        'There may be some role for medical treatments such as laxatives.'

Educational

'We will aim to educate yourself and your child about the problem and what can be done. We can begin keeping a stool diary.'

Psychological

Family therapy

Social/behavioural interventions

'We can use different behavioural techniques, such as sitting the child on the toilet for up to five minutes three or four times a day post meals and using a reward system, to help to reinforce defaecation in the toilet or urination in the toilet.'

Prognosis

Good

Most will completely recover (>75%)

REFERENCES

Gowers, S. (ed.). *College Seminars Series: Seminars in Child and Adolescent Psychiatry*, (2nd edn) (2005) Royal College of Psychiatrists pp. 28–39

Goodman, R. & Scott, S. *Child Psychiatry* (2nd edn) Blackwell pp. 126–136

CONDUCT DISORDER

Core diagnostic criteria (ICD-10)

Types of conduct disorder
- Family context, only in the family context
- Oppositional defiant disorder, less antisocial behaviour
- Socialised, popular with peers
- Unsocialised, unpopular with peers

Key phrases

'What difficulties has Johnny been having?'
'How long has this been going on for?' (needs to be six months)
'Has he ever been in trouble with the law?'
'Has he ever broken the law that you know of?'
'Does he have many friends?'
'Is he the same at home and at school?'
'Can you think of any possible trigger for this?'
'Does he have any physical illnesses?'
'Ever had a seizure?'

Features
- 'Does he have temper tantrums?'
- 'Does he often argue with adults?'
- 'Does he refuse requests or break rules?'
- "Does he try to annoy others?'
- 'Does he blame others for his mistakes?'
- 'Would you say he is easily annoyed?'
- 'Do you think he is angry?'
- 'Would you say he was spiteful or vindictive?'
- 'Does he ever lie or break promises?'
- 'Does he fight with those other than his siblings?'
- 'Has he ever used a weapon?'
- 'Has he ever stayed out after dark?'
- 'Has he ever been physically cruel to anyone?'
- 'Has he ever been physically cruel to animals?'
- 'Has he ever destroyed property?'
- 'Has he ever started a fire?'
- 'Does he ever steal things?'
- 'Has he played truant from school?'
- 'Has he ever run away from home?'
- 'Has he ever stolen from someone's person?'
- 'Has he ever forced anyone into a sexual act?'
- 'Would you say he is a bully?'
- 'Has he ever broken into a car or a building?'

General
- 'Can you think of anything else I should know about?'
- 'How do you cope?'
- 'What effect is this having on the family?'

Don't forget symptoms of ADHD and other mental illnesses

Information giving

Oppositional Defiant Disorder is generally in younger children who do not display the more
extreme forms of aggression or dissocial behaviour
Management
Behavioural approach
Parent training/education programmes (NICE)
Family therapy

Essential guidelines (NICE guidelines on conduct disorder 2007)

Recommend group based parent training/education programmes unless needs too complicated
or difficult to engage then use individual training
Usually 8–12 sessions

REFERENCES

Gowers, S. (ed.). *College Seminars Series: Seminars in Child and Adolescent Psychiatry,* (2nd edn) (2005) Royal College
of Psychiatrists pp. 145–158
Goodman, R. & Scott, S. *Child Psychiatry,* (2nd edn) Blackwell pp. 59–69
NICE Clinical Guidelines (2006) *Parent-training/education programmes in the management of children with conduct
disorders.* National Institute for Clinical Excellence
Cooper, J. (ed.).(2004) *Pocket Guide to the ICD-10: Classification of Mental and Behavioural Disorders.* Churchill
Livingstone pp. 289–325

3.5 SUBSTANCE MISUSE

ALCOHOL (DEPENDENCE, DETOXIFICATION, HISTORY, HAZARDS, AND EXAMINATION)

Alcohol dependence

Core diagnostic criteria (ICD-10)

Dependence syndrome (three or more for one month constant or 12 months intermittent)
  Compulsion
  Poor control
  Withdrawal
  Tolerance
  Primacy
  Persistence despite harm

Key phrases

Confirming dependence (ICD-10)
  Subjective awareness of a compulsion to drink
    'Do you feel you must drink?'
  Poor control
    'Are you able to control how much you drink?'
    'Can you control when you drink?'
  Repeated withdrawal symptoms
    'What happens if you don't drink?'
    'When you are feeling like that, what are you thinking about?'
    'If you then take a drink, how does it make you feel?'
  Altered tolerance
    'How much do you drink per day?'
    'Have you always drunk this amount?'
    'Do you find that you need to drink more than you used to in order to get the same effect?'
  Primacy of drinking over other activities
    'What do you do in your spare time?'
    'Did you use to do other things?'
    'Do you feel alcohol has stopped you doing certain things?'
  Persistence despite harm
    'Have you ever had difficulties because of your drinking?'
    'Has drinking ever affected your physical health?'
    'Why do you think you have continued to drink in spite of this?'
Others (Edwards & Gross 1976)
  Narrowing of drinking repertoire
    'What do you drink?'
    'Did you use to drink other drinks as well?'
  Rapid reinstatement after abstinence
    'Have you ever tried to give up alcohol?'
    'How long did you manage to give up alcohol?'

Alcohol detoxification

Information giving

Motivation

'Are you interested in giving up alcohol?'

'Have you had any treatments before?'

'What did that involve?'

Explanation

'I understand that you are interested in alcohol detoxification. We can do this either in the community or as an inpatient.'

'The choice of treatment setting depends on a number of factors such as your physical and mental health, your blood test results, and whether there is a responsible adult who could stay with you during a home detox. If you have a history of certain physical illnesses such as seizures, or a history of serious mental illness, an inpatient detox would probably be the safer option.'

'In either case we use "symptom triggered" treatment with drugs called benzodiazepines which work by relieving withdrawal symptoms. This involves a nurse assessing you for withdrawal symptoms every 90 minutes to make sure you receive the appropriate dose of the benzodiazepine medication. We usually use a drug called diazepam. This will continue until you have no further withdrawal symptoms.'

'We also recommend thiamine, which is a kind of Vitamin B. It is given as a tablet or sometimes by injection, depending on your risk of deficiency. A multivitamin tablet or injection is often also given just before you start the detox. The vitamins are usually continued for at least a month.'

'A tablet by the name of acamprosate (Campral) may also be prescribed just before your detox to help decrease your craving for alcohol. This may also protect you from nerve damage.'

'A detox is usually the beginning of a long journey to complete recovery. We may also recommend a tablet called disulfiram (Antabuse) to help you stay off the alcohol. This tablet is taken daily and if you drink alcohol whilst you are taking these tablets, you will experience a series of unpleasant reactions. It is given as a deterrent to alcohol use.'

'After the acute phase, a period of rehabilitation is sometimes appropriate. This very much depends on the severity of your drinking and your social circumstances, such as your family and work.'

'Rehabilitation can be for a period of up to six months or even longer.'

'The rehabilitation unit provides an environment of individual and group sessions to strengthen coping mechanisms in dealing with alcohol.'

'Rehabilitation occurs in a drug- and alcohol-free environment.'

Alcohol history

Key phrases

First alcoholic drink

'How old were you when you had your first alcoholic drink?'

'What sort of drink was it?'

Drinking pattern

'When do you start drinking each day?'

'Do you ever have a drink in the morning?'

If the patient drinks daily

'Have you always drunk alcohol on a daily basis?'
'When did you start drinking more?'
'Was the increase gradual?'
'What would happen if you weren't to have a drink?'
Assessing the impact of the alcohol use
  Social
    'Has drinking alcohol ever affected your relationships with friends and family?'
    'Have you ever missed work because of alcohol?'
    'Have you ever lost a job because of alcohol?'
    'Has drinking alcohol ever affected the way you spend your free time?'
  Physical health
    'Have you had any physical symptoms since drinking this much?'
    'Sometimes people who drink a lot of alcohol get things like stomach ulcers. Have you ever had anything like that?'
    'Have you ever had a fit or a seizure?'
    'Have you ever had delirium tremens or "DTs"? This is when people get extremely unwell, may be drowsy and may see things that other people cannot see or that may not be there?'
  Mental health
    'How is your mood?'
    'Tell me about your sleep.'
    'How is your appetite?'
    'Are you able to concentrate?'
    'Have things ever got that bad that you felt like harming yourself?'
  Family history
    'Has anyone in your family ever had any problems with alcohol?'
  Financial
    'Are you in any financial difficulties because of the amount of alcohol you drink?'
  Forensic
    'Have you ever been in trouble with the police?'
    'Have you ever had any driving offences or offences related to drinking such as drunk and disorderly?'

Alcohol hazards

Information giving

Find out what patient already knows
  'Are you aware of the problems related to drinking alcohol?'
Biological
  Gastrointestinal
    Gastritis
    Peptic ulcer (10%)
    Pancreatitis
    Gastrointestinal bleeds due to tears or varices
  Liver disease
    Fat deposition/cirrhosis
    Treatments are not very successful but transplantation is an option
  Cardiovascular
    Hypertension
    CVA
    Cardiac arrhythmias

Sexual impairment
    Erectile dysfunction
    Loss of libido
Neurological: Wernicke's encephalopathy
    (C)   Confusion/clouding of consciousness
    (A)   Ataxia
    (N)   Nystagmus
    (O)   Ophthalmoplegia
    (N)   Neuropathy
Congenital impairment
    Foetal alcohol syndrome
Psychiatric
    Delirium tremens ('DTs')
        Tremor
        Clouding of consciousness
        Fever
        Sweating
        Tachycardia
        Mortality is around 10%
    Alcoholic hallucinosis
        Hallucinations in clear consciousness
    Korsakoff's psychosis
        Short-term memory impairment
        Peripheral neuropathy
        Late-onset
        Total recovery is rare
    Depression
    Anxiety
Social
    Employment problems
    Financial difficulties
    Disruption of family relationships
    Accidents and offences due to being drunk

Driving
Alcohol dependency
    Before being able to drive, person must be free of alcohol problems for one year and blood
    parameters must be normal
Alcohol misuse
    Before being able to drive, person must have demonstrated six months of controlled drinking

Alcohol examination
Appropriate exposure
Global
    Pallor
    Jaundice
    Loss of body hair
Hands
    Palmar erythema
    Clubbing
    Dupuytren's contracture

Xanthomas (look in palmar creases)
Liver flap (hepatic encephalopathy)

Eyes
    Jaundice
    Xanthelasmas

Head
    Parotid enlargement
    Fetor hepaticus

Thorax
    Spider naevi or telangiectases (look above nipple line)
    Gynaecomastia

Abdomen
    Hepatomegaly (or small liver later)
    Splenomegaly
    Ascites
    Scratch marks
    Dilated veins on abdomen (caput medusae – very rare)

Neurological
    Global
        Disorientation
        Drowsiness
    Cerebellar signs
        (D)   Dysdiadochokinesia
        (A)   Ataxia
        (N)   Nystagmus
        (I)   Intentional tremor
        (S)   Slurred speech
        (H)   Hypotonia
    Sensory signs
        Glove and stocking sensory impairment (tingling or numbness)
    Motor signs
        Muscle wasting
        Decreased power

Genital
    Testicular atrophy

Legs
    Purpura
    Pigmented ulcers
    Pedal and ankle oedema

REFERENCES

Cooper, J. (ed.) (2004). *Pocket Guide to the ICD-10: Classification of Mental and Behavioural Disorders.* Churchill Livingstone pp 63–91

Chick, J. & Cantwell, R. (ed.) (1994). *College Seminars Series: Seminars in Alcohol and Drug Misuse.* Royal College of Psychiatrists pp. 1–17

Gelder, M., Harrison, P. & Cowen, P. (2001). *Shorter Oxford Textbook of Psychiatry* (5th edn) Oxford University Press pp. 429–450

DRUG MISUSE (OPIATES, COCAINE, AMPHETAMINE, CANNABIS, MDMA)

Key phrases

Details
  'What drugs do you take?'
  'In what form do you take them?'
  'How do you take them?'
  'How long have you been using them?'
Determining dependence (e.g. heroin)
  Compulsion
    'Do you feel compelled to use heroin?'
  Poor control
    'Are you able to control how much you take?'
    'Are you able to control when you take it?'
  Repeated withdrawal symptoms
    'What happens if you don't take heroin?'
    'When you are feeling like that, what are you thinking about?'
    'When you take heroin again, how do you then feel?'
  Altered tolerance
    'How much heroin do you use per week?'
    'Have you always taken this amount?'
    'Do you find that you need to take more than you used to in order to get the same effect?'
  Primacy of drug-taking over other activities
    'What do you do in your spare time?'
    'Did you use to do other things?'
    'Do you feel using heroin has stopped you doing certain things?'
  Persistence despite harm
    'Have you ever had any difficulties due to your drug taking?'
    'Why do you think you have continued to take heroin in spite of this?'
    'Has using drugs ever affected your physical health, such as getting an abscess around a needle site or contracting a disease such as hepatitis?'

Information giving

Management options
  Determining motivation
    'What made you want to seek help?'
    'What benefits do you see by giving up drugs?'
  Harm minimization model
    'It is important to use clean needles and syringes when injecting drugs such as heroin. This will reduce your risk of contracting diseases like HIV and hepatitis B and C.'
    'We can teach you safe injection techniques to reduce the risk of complications such as injecting air into your bloodstream.'
    'One way to use heroin more safely is to insert it into your back passage. There is good blood supply to this part of the body and so heroin is easily absorbed from here. This is an option to think about, especially if you cannot find a suitable vein.'
    'Safe sex is very important for everyone, but because certain infections are more common in people who inject drugs such as heroin, it is important that you consider using a condom as a preventative measure.'

'Addiction services are here to help you and so it is important that you stay in regular contact.'

Short-term

Symptomatic treatment of withdrawal (especially for opiates)

Nausea: Metoclopramide 10mg tds

Abdominal cramps: Hyoscine butylbromide (Buscopan) 20mg qds

Diarrhoea: Loperamide 4mg stat then 2mg after every loose motion

Muscle and joint pain/headaches: Ibuprofen 400—600mg tds

Anxiety/agitation: Diazepam 5mg qds

General symptoms (including sweats, chills, runny nose): Lofexidine (BritLofex) 0.2mg tablets up to 2.4mg/day

Substitute therapy

Methadone, an opioid agonist

Buprenorphine (Subutex), an opioid partial agonist

Substitute prescribing

Aim is to stabilize patient on the substitute medication (methadone or buprenorphine) to help them make the necessary changes to their lifestyle (e.g. change circle of friends, settle at home, re-connect with family) before they start their detox.

Methadone or buprenorphine can be initiated in outpatient clinic. The choice of treatment setting mainly depends on the patient's own preference but some important clinical factors such as level of drug use, risk of overdose and respiratory depression may make treatment in an inpatient setting a safer option.. Before initiating treatment important to confirm dependence by at least three drug serial urine drug screens.

Opiate detoxification (four weeks inpatient or 12 weeks community)

Detox can be done in community or in-patient setting. Various regimes of detox can be used such as slow methadone or buprenorphine withdrawal in the community, change over to buprenorphine and then withdrawal, quick buprenorphine in-patient detox or lofexidine assisted detox.

Long term maintenance treatment

Some people may need long term treatment with methadone or buprenorphine. This can be done with regular follow up in the community.

Long term treatment after detox

Rehabilitation programs are available funded by social services.

Relapse prevention programmes and counselling is useful.

Contingency management such as vouchers to promote abstinence

Naltrexone, an opioid antagonist used to maintain abstinence.

Driving

Heroin, methadone, methamphetamine or cocaine

Before being able to drive, person must be free from drug for one year

Cannabis, amphetamine, ecstasy or LSD

Before being able to drive, person must be free from drug for six months

Essential guidelines (NICE guidelines 2007)

Decide between methadone and buprenorphine on a case by case basis and if equally suitable use methadone.

Can use naltrexone in those who are detoxified and highly motivated to stay in an abstinence programme.

REFERENCES

Cooper, J. (ed.).(2004) *Pocket Guide to the ICD-10: Classification of Mental and Behavioural Disorders.* Churchill Livingstone pp. 63–91

Jarvis et al. *Treatment approaches for alcohol and drug dependence, an introductory guide.* (2nd edn) (2005) John Wiley & Sons pp.193–207

Chick, J. & Cantwell, R. (ed.).(1994) *College Seminars Series: Seminars in Alcohol and Drug Misuse.* Royal College of Psychiatrists pp. 19–32

Joint Formulary Committee. British National Formulary. (56th edn) (2008) British Medical Association and Royal Pharmaceutical Society of Great Britain pp. 266–271

NICE Clinical Guidelines (2007) *Drug Misuse.* National Institute for Clinical Excellence

NICE Clinical Guidelines (2007) *Naltrexone for the management of opioid dependence.* National Institute for Clinical Excellence

NICE Clinical Guidelines (2007) *Methadone and buprenorphine for the management of opioid dependence.* National Institute for Clinical Excellence

OPIOID USE IN PREGNANCY

Key phrases

'When did you first realise you were pregnant?'
'Is this your first pregnancy?'
'Have you had any scans or tests so far?'
'How much heroin are you using?'

Information giving

'All pregnant women should be tested for HIV and hepatitis B and C.'
'Social services will not be automatically notified. They only become involved if there are any concerns for your baby's safety or you need some extra help.'
'Methadone is ok to use in pregnancy and has been used for a long time. Subutex is a much newer drug and therefore less pregnant women have used it. There is a suggestion that it causes fewer withdrawal symptoms in babies.'
'There is no evidence that methadone or heroin causes abnormalities but there is slight risk of prematurity or having a small baby.'
'Risks are reduced if you are on prescribed medication, attend appointments regularly and look after your own health.'
'If you overdose, your baby may die, and you may die.'
'If you have bad withdrawal symptoms then your baby will have withdrawal symptoms and there is a risk of miscarriage or premature birth.'
'We advise the avoidance of alcohol, all street drugs, especially cocaine, and benzodiazepines such as diazepam which is also called Valium.'
'We can help you to detox at any time but it must be slow. You can have paracetamol, loperamide and sleeping tablets but not aspirin or ibuprofen.'
'It is way safer to be on a stable dose of methadone than withdraw or use street heroin.'
'During labour we have to be careful with pain relief. We recommend gas and air or an epidural. Other drugs can be used be we have to be very cautious.'
'You will continue your replacement therapy throughout labour and the birth.'
'After the birth the baby may withdraw. He will be monitored with you in hospital for five days. If your baby shows any signs of withdrawal he may have to stay longer. Some babies may need to have small doses of sedatives to help them through the withdrawal.'
'You can breast feed if you are on less than 80mls methadone and are not taking street drugs.'
'We are here to help you every step of the way and are really pleased that you have been honest with us and sought help.'

REFERENCES

Heroin and other opiates in pregnancy Patient information leaflet for the Gloucester Health Community.

SMOKING CESSATION

Key phrases

'How much are you smoking?'
'Why do you want to give up?'
'Do you think this is the right time in your life to give up smoking?'
'Have you tried to give up before?'
'What happened?'
'Are you taking any other substances?'
'How is your general health at the moment?'

Information giving

'Motivation is essential for success'.
Assessing motivation (stages of change)
    Precontemplation
        No intent to change behaviour in the near future
    Contemplation
        Openly state their intent to change within the next six months
    Preparation
        Intend to take steps to change, usually within the next month
    Action
        Has made overt, perceptible lifestyle modifications for less than months
    Maintenance
        Working to prevent relapse and consolidate gains
General
    Set a date to quit and get rid of all smoking paraphernalia
    Inform people around him and enlist their support
    If has a partner are they going to quit too?
    Encourage to cut down intake before starting to quit
    Discuss benefits of stopping e.g. health, finances
    Inform will be difficult and may relapse
    Look at possible relapse triggers
    Possibility of withdrawal symptoms
    Possibility of weight gain but only 10% have significant weight increases
    Refer to local smoking cessation clinic
Medical Treatment
    Nicotine replacement therapy (NRT)
        Nasal sprays, patches, chewing gum, lozenges, inhalers, sublingual tablets
        Dose dependent of how much is smoking
        Gradual withdrawal
        Discontinue if relapse
        Side effects: localised irritation, sleep disturbances
    Bupropion (Zyban)
        Weak re-uptake inhibitor of dopamine and noradrenalin
        150mg for six days then 300mg from day six to eight weeks (max 12 weeks). Stop
        smoking after 7–14 days .
        Need to rule out epilepsy or seizures and hepatic problems
        Side effects: seizures (1 in 1000), sensitivity reactions such as bronchospasm (1 in 1000),
        rash, dry mouth, weight loss, insomnia, rarely cardiac problems
    Antidepressants e.g. nortryptiline or amitryptiline
        Evidence not great

Naltrexone (opioid antagonist)
    May reduce amount smoked but evidence not great
Varenicline (Champix)
    Nicotinic receptor partial agonist
    0.5mg od days 1–3, 0.5mg bd days 4–7, 1mg bd day eight to 12 weeks
    Can have further weeks if have achieved abstinence
    Need to rule out kidney problems, depression, and epilepsy
    Side effects: depression, insomnia, dizziness, sleepiness, headache, dry mouth
Effectiveness
    Placebo = 10%, NRT = 17%, Bupropion = 20%, Varenicline = 20%
    Need to consider if has any mental illness and how this may impact

Essential guidelines (NICE guidelines on smoking cessation 2002, NICE guidelines on Varenicline 2007)

The NHS will in usual circumstances fund one attempt to quit smoking per six months
There is no evidence that Bupropion and NRT together improve quit rates
Varenicline is a suitable drug of choice for smoking cessation

REFERENCES

Joint Formulary Committee. *British National Formulary*. (56th edn) (2008) British Medical Association and Royal Pharmaceutical Society of Great Britain pp. 266–271
NICE Clinical Guidelines (2007) *Varenicline for smoking cessation*. National Institute for Clinical Excellence
NICE Clinical Guidelines (2002) *Guidance on the use of nicotine replacement therapy (NRT) and bupropion for smoking cessation*. National Institute for Clinical Excellence

DISSOCIAL PERSONALITY DISORDER

Core diagnostic criteria (ICD-10)

The general criteria for personality disorder must be met, and at least three of the following must be present:
- (I)   Incapacity to maintain enduring relationships
- (T)   Tends to blame others
- (A)   Attitude of irresponsibility and disregard for social norms and rules
- (L)   Low tolerance to frustration and low threshold for discharge of aggression
- (I)   Incapacity to experience guilt, or to profit from adverse experience
- (C)   Callous unconcern for the feelings of others

Key phrases

In practice much of the information that is needed to make a diagnosis of dissocial personality disorder is gathered from historical notes and collateral history. However, the following history taking key phrases will show the examiner that you are familiar with the core diagnostic criteria.

Incapacity to maintain enduring relationships (though with no difficulty in establishing them)
   'Tell me about your relationships?'
   'How many have you had?'
Tends to blame others
   'Do you think that anyone else may be to blame for things that have happened to you?'
Attitude of irresponsibility and disregard for social norms and rules
   'Do you ever find it difficult to abide by rules?'
   'Do you find it hard to stay out of trouble?'
   'Do you ever take chances and do reckless things?'
Low tolerance to frustration and low threshold for discharge of aggression
   'Do you lose your temper easily?'
   'Have you been involved in many fights or arguments?'
Incapacity to experience guilt, or to profit from adverse experience
   'Have you ever spent time in prison or been in trouble with the law?'
   'How did this make you feel?'
Callous unconcern for the feelings of others
   'How do you respond if others are frightened or upset?'
Extras
   Persistent irritability
      'Are you easily irritated?'
   Conduct disorder during childhood or adolescence
      'How did you get on at school? Were you often in trouble with other children or the teachers?'
   Co-morbid conditions
      Mood disorders, anxiety disorders, substance misuse, eating disorders, psychosis, post-traumatic stress disorder
   Current functioning
      Enquire about work/education, social, intimate relationships, sex life
   Risk of harm to others
      'Have you ever harmed anyone else?'
      'Have you ever been in trouble with the law?'
      'Is there anyone you wish to come to harm?'

Information giving

Explain diagnosis

'The pattern of how we tend to deal with situations and how we think about ourselves and interact with others makes up our personality. If the way someone tends to deal with things causes significant problems or is upsetting or distressing, then it is possible they may have personality difficulties or be diagnosed as having a personality disorder. Many of the difficulties you have described such as ... have been present since childhood, and are best understood as part of your personality. The clinical term for this is dissocial personality disorder.'

'People who have dissocial personality disorder often have problems in understanding the feelings of others, and may experience difficulties with taking responsibility for their actions.'

'Although people with dissocial personality disorder might not have any problems with forming relationships, they often find it difficult to maintain them.'

'You may also find that you lose your temper easily, and sometimes you may feel like hitting out.'

Treatment

The evidence base for the treatment of dissocial personality disorder is limited (see below).

Essential Guidelines (NICE guidelines antisocial personality disorder 2009)

Psychological

Group-based cognitive and behavioural interventions to address problems such as impulsivity, interpersonal difficulties and antisocial behaviour.

In people with a history of offending, interventions should be focussed on reducing offending and other antisocial behaviour, they include cognitive behavioural programmes such as Reasoning and Rehabilitation and Enhanced Thinking Skills.

Pharmacological

Medication should not be routinely used for the treatment of antisocial personality disorder or associated behaviours of aggression, anger and impulsivity. Medication should be considered for co-morbid mental disorders as appropriate.

REFERENCES

Cooper, J. (ed.).(2004) *Pocket Guide to the ICD-10: Classification of Mental and Behavioural Disorders*. Churchill Livingstone pp. 226–228

NICE Clinical Guidelines (2009) *Antisocial personality disorder: treatment, management and prevention*. National Institute for Clinical Excellence

Tong, L.S.J. & Farrington, D.P. (2006). *How effective is the 'Reasoning and Rehabilitation' programme in reducing reoffending? A meta-analysis of evaluations in four countries*. Psychology, Crime & Law, **12**(1), 3–24

SEXUAL OFFENDING (PSYCHOSEXUAL HISTORY, PARAPHILIAS AND MANAGEMENT)

Psychosexual history (from a male)

Key phrases

Introduction

'I'd like to ask you about your sex life. Some of the questions I need to ask you are very personal but they are the same questions I have to ask everyone. I don't wish to offend you and so if any of the questions sound strange please do not feel insulted.'

Puberty and adolescence

'How did you first learn about sex?'

'What age were you when you started puberty?'

'Do you remember having wet dreams?'

'How old were you when you started masturbating?'

'How regularly did you masturbate?'

'When did you have your first kiss?',

'Did it lead on to anything else?'

'When did you have your first sexual encounter?'

'When did you lose your virginity?',

'Who was it with?',

'Did you want to lose it at that time?',

'Did you feel pushed into it?'

Other sexual encounters

'Can you give me an idea of how many sexual partners you have had?'

'Have you ever had unprotected sex?'

'Have you ever pushed anyone into sleeping with you?'

'Has anyone ever accused you of forcing them to have sex?'

'Have you ever paid anyone to have sex?'

'Have you ever had a sexual experience with a man?'

'With children?'

Current sexual health

'How is your sex life?'

'How often do you have sex?'

'Is there any tension between you and your [wife/partner] about this?'

'Have you ever had an affair?'

'Do you ever have a problem getting an erection?'

Fantasies and pornography

'When you started masturbating, did you used to masturbate to a fantasy?'

'What was the fantasy?'

'Have you ever had any fantasies about sexual contact with men?'

'Have you ever been sexually excited by children'

'Have you ever had a fantasy where you were in charge of a sexual partner?'

'Has this ever involved violence?'

'Have you ever fantasised about taking someone by force?'

'Have you ever used pornography?'

'What sort of pornography do you use?'

'Have you ever used violent pornography?'

'Have you ever used child pornography?'

Screening for disorders of sexual preference (the paraphilias)

Core diagnostic criteria (ICD-10)

The following criteria are general to all disorders of sexual preference:

The individual experiences recurrent intense sexual urges and fantasies involving unusual objects or activities

The individual either acts on the urges or is markedly distressed by them

The preference has been present for at least six months

For each disorder of sexual preference, see the Key phrases section below. For the specific criteria please refer to an ICD-10 manual.

Key phrases

F65.0 Fetishism

'Have you ever been sexually excited by objects such as shoes?'

'Do you have to use/imagine them to reach orgasm?'

F65.1 Fetishistic transvestism

'Have you ever dressed in women's clothing?'

'Was it for sexual excitement?'

In fetishistic transvestism, once orgasm occurs; there is a strong desire to remove the clothing

F65.2 Exhibitionism

'Have you ever exposed yourself in public?'

'Who did/do you expose yourself to?'

'Where did/do you do it?'

'How often did/do you do it?'

'Was/is it sexually exciting for you?'

'Did/do you masturbate whilst doing it?'

In exhibitionism, there is no intention of sexual involvement with the victim

F65.3 Voyeurism

'Have you ever felt the urge to watch others undressing or while they are having sexual intercourse?'

In voyeurism, there is no intention of sexual involvement with the victim

F65.4 Paedophilia

'Have you ever been sexually attracted to children?'

'How old is he?'

'How long did this last, are you still doing this?'

Others

F65.5 Sadomasochism (must involve pain, humiliation or bondage)

'Have you ever needed to use bondage to reach orgasm?'

'Is receiving or causing pain sexually exciting for you?'

F65.8 Other disorders of sexual preference (includes frotteurism and necrophilia)

'Have you ever made obscene phone-calls?'

'Have you ever followed anyone?'

Management of sex offenders

Cognitive Bahaviour Therapy (CBT)

The essential components (STEP report 1994)

Discuss offence cycle

Challenge cognitive distortions

Victim empathy

Fantasy modification

Social skills and anger control

Relapse prevention

The sex offender treatment programme (SOTP)

The SOTP is available in certain prisons and hospitals and it is based on the CBT model. It is not suitable for offenders with a mental illness. There are four parts to the SOTP:

The core programme

The thinking skills programme

The extended programme

The relapse prevention programme

Pharmacological treatment (anti-libidinals)

Anti-libidinals work by reducing testosterone levels. Reducing testosterone levels is thought to reduce the rates of sexual offending.

The medications:

Anti-androgens e.g. cyproterone acetate

Gonadorelin analogues e.g. triptorelin

Psychoanalytic psychotherapy and behavioural therapy

Psychoanalytic psychotherapy was seen as the most effective treatment of sex offenders before CBT. However most outcome studies show it is ineffective, and some studies which report higher rates of recidivism.

REFERENCES

Cooper, J. (ed.). (2004) *Pocket Guide to the ICD-10: Classification of Mental and Behavioural Disorders.* Churchill Livingstone pp. 249–254

Gelder, M., Harrison, P. & Cowen, P. (2001). *Shorter Oxford Textbook of Psychiatry* (5th edn) Oxford University Press pp. 314–316 & 471–494

Gordon, H. & Grubin, D. (2004). Psychiatric aspects of the assessment and treatment of sex offenders *Advances in Psychiatric Treatment* **10**, 73–80.

Stone, J.H., Roberts, M., O'Grady & J., Taylor, A.V. (ed.).(2000) *Faulk's Basic Forensic Psychiatry* (3rd edn) Blackwell pp. 223–230

PATHOLOGICAL JEALOUSY

Core information

As pathological jealousy is not a diagnosis in its own right, it follows that there are no set diagnostic criteria.

Key feature
  Abnormal belief in a partner's infidelity (may be a delusion or an overvalued idea)
Other clinical features
  Intensive seeking for evidence of the infidelity
  Disturbed mood
Can arise from
  Mood disorders
  Schizophrenia
  Delusional disorders
  Substance misuse (including alcohol)
  Organic disorders (including learning disability & dementia)

Key phrases

To confirm seeking for evidence
  'Have you ever followed your partner?'
  'Have you ever followed the person you think they're having an affair with?'
  'Have you ever thought about hiring a detective to spy on them?'
To establish delusional belief/overvalued idea
  'Have you ever seen them together?'
  'Were they kissing?'
  'Did you catch them in bed?'
  'So how do you know?'
  'Then how do you know she's having an affair?'
  'Have you ever seen any signs to prove it's going on?'
  'How does that prove they're having an affair?'
  'Have you ever confronted her about it?'
  'What did she say?'
  'Do you think she might have just confessed because she just did not know what else to say?'
  In delusional jealousy, forced false confessions may inflame the situation
Risk of violence to partner (a quarter of individuals threaten to kill or injure their partner)
  'How has all this made you feel?'
  'Have you ever had any arguments or fights with your partner over this?'
  'Have you ever come to blows?'
  'Tell me what happened'
  'How often has it happened?'
  'Have you ever physically injured your partner during a fight?'
  'Have you ever felt like harming your partner?'
  'How close were you?'
  'Have you ever had any thoughts of taking your partner's life because of this?'
Risk of violence to supposed rival (around half threaten to kill or injure the supposed rival)
  'Have you ever wanted to harm the man you think your partner is seeing?'
  'Have you ever thought how you might go about this?'
  'Do you carry a weapon?'
  'What do you do for a living?'
  'What if you got the wrong man?'

Risk of self-harm
'Has all of this ever made you want to harm yourself?'
'What have you been thinking about doing?'
Risk to children
'Do you have any children?'
'If you were to end it all what would happen to the children?'

Information giving

Treatment
Treat comorbidity (e.g. substance misuse)
Medication
Antipsychotics for delusions
SSRIs (when jealousy is an overvalued idea)
Psychotherapy
CBT
Couple therapy
Individual dynamic psychotherapy (especially in personality disorders where borderline and paranoid traits are present)
Risk management
If there is risk of violence, the partner should be informed even if this involves a breach of confidentiality
If delusional jealousy is resistant to treatment then geographical separation of the partners may be necessary
Liaise with MAPPA (Multi-Agency Public Protection Arrangements)
Even if the jealousy wanes when the relationship ends, there is a risk of it re-emerging in a future relationship

REFERENCES

Stone, J.H., Roberts, M., O'Grady, J. & Taylor, A.V. (eds) (2000). *Faulk's Basic Forensic Psychiatry* (3rd edn) Blackwell pp. 150–151

Gelder, M., Harrison, P. & Cowen, P. (2001). *Shorter Oxford Textbook of Psychiatry* (5th edn) Oxford University Press pp. 314–316

Kingham, M. & Gordon, H. (2004). Aspects of morbid jealousy. *Advances in Psychiatric Treatment*, **10**, 207–215

FORENSIC PSYCHIATRY AND THE LAW (FITNESS TO PLEAD, PSYCHIATRIC DEFENCES, FORENSIC SECTIONS, WRITING A COURT REPORT)

Fitness to plead (Pritchard Rules)

Core information

This question may be raised by the defence, the prosecution or the judge. An impairment of any of the following would suggest that the defendant is unfit to plead:

To understand the charge and its implications

'What do you understand that you have been accused of?'

Able to instruct counsel

'What is the role of a lawyer?'

Understand plea and implications

'What is a plea?'

'What does guilty mean?'

'What would pleading guilty mean?'

To comprehend the course of the proceedings of the trial

'Do you know what happens in a criminal trial?'

To know that he might challenge a juror

'What is the role of a jury?'

'Do you understand that you have the right to ask for a different jury or a different juror if you believe the jury has been selected unfairly, or if you believe that the juror is biased or unqualified to be a juror?'

To comprehend the details of the evidence

'How is evidence used in a criminal trial?'

The psychiatric defences

Core information

Not guilty by reason of insanity (NGRI or the 'special verdict')

The accused must prove that at the time of committing the act he was of diseased mind and that

He did not know the nature/quality of the act

or if he did know it, he did not know that it was wrong

Infanticide

This defence may be used by a woman who is charged with the murder of her child who is 12 months or younger. It may also be the primary charge.

It must be proven that 'the balance of mind was disturbed' as a result of the effects of birth or lactation.

Diminished responsibility

This defence can only be used if the charge is murder.

The defendant must demonstrate that he was suffering from an abnormality of mind which substantially impaired his mental responsibility for the killing.

Automatism

The defendant claims he was acting 'automatically' or in other words the defendant is not conscious of what he is doing.

Non-insane automatism (due to external causes e.g. blow to the head)

Insane automatism (due to internal causes e.g. epilepsy)

Mentally disordered offenders and the Mental Health Act

Core information

The Mental Health Act makes the following provisions for mentally disordered offenders:

35 To remand the accused to hospital for psychiatric reports

36 To remand the accused to hospital for treatment

37 To order the convicted to go to hospital for treatment

38 The order the convicted to go to hospital to 'trial treatment' (known as the interim hospital order)

47 To transfer a sentenced prisoner to hospital

48 To transfer a remanded prisoner to hospital

41 To restrict a patient subject to Section 37
    (Leave outside hospital and discharge can only be granted by secretary of State)

49 To restrict a sentenced prisoner subject to Sections 47/48
    (This restriction order expires at the prisoner's earliest release date)

Writing a psychiatric report for criminal proceedings

Core information

In this situation, it is important to remember the following

Check personal details
    Rarely the wrong prisoner is produced for interview.

State the purpose of the interview
    'The purpose of this interview is to.'

Explain that the report will not be confidential
    'I have been instructed by X to prepare a report for the court. Our discussion today is therefore not confidential as it is when you normally speak to your own doctor.'
    'It is likely that my report will be read by other people involved in your legal case, and maybe heard in court.'

Remember that a remanded prisoner has not been convicted so keep language neutral
    'You have been charged with....'

REFERENCES

Gunn, J. & Taylor, P.J. (eds) (1993) *Forensic Psychiatry: Clinical, Legal & Ethical Issues.* Butterworth Heinemann. pp. 21–118

Chiswick, D. & Cope, R. (ed.) (1998). *College Seminars Series: Seminars in Practical Forensic Psychiatry.* The Royal College of Psychiatrists pp.138–139

COGNITIVE BEHAVIOURAL THERAPY (CBT)

Description

'CBT stands for Cognitive Behavioural Therapy and it is a kind of talking therapy. It has a strong evidence base for effectiveness in many mental disorders.'

'CBT has been found to be helpful in several conditions such as depression, anxiety, phobias, obsessive compulsive disorder and bulimia. It can also be helpful with psychotic conditions such as schizophrenia.'

'CBT uses a model in which thinking, feelings and actions are all seen as linked and connected.'

'CBT helps to improve symptoms by identifying and exploring how certain negative thinking patterns and behaviours can make people vulnerable to feeling bad about themselves, the world and the future. By challenging these negative thinking patterns, they can begin to feel more in control of their lives, and more optimistic about themselves.'

'During CBT patients also learn techniques to help them solve problems themselves, so that in the future they will be able to tackle problems without the help of a therapist.'

How it works

CBT may be given one to one or within a group setting. It may also be accessed on the computer.

The therapist and the patient will usually meet every week or fortnight. The number of sessions each person needs varies, but usually the therapy will last between 5–20 sessions. Each session usually lasts between 30 minutes and an hour.

You don't have to stop taking medication to receive CBT. It is often helpful to have both together.

Key terms

Negative automatic thoughts

When people are depressed or anxious they tend to see themselves and the world in a more negative light. Their low mood makes it more likely that they will remember sad or distressing memories rather than happy or positive ones. If they are anxious they may misperceive internal and external cues as more threatening or frightening than they are.

CBT helps a person to identify these negative thoughts and behaviour patterns, which may be feeding into a vicious cycle.

CBT helps a person to start to challenge these thoughts and work out different ways to think and behave.

Practical steps

CBT often involves doing homework between sessions, such as keeping a mood diary; scheduling activities through the day; and learning to recognise thinking errors.

Rules for living

CBT can also help people to look at their 'rules for living.' These are strong beliefs about how we should live our lives. CBT helps us to become aware of these rules and develop rules that are more helpful.

Here and now

CBT focuses primarily on the 'here and now' rather than issues from the past.

Schemas

More recently CBT work involving 'schemas' has been developed for people with longer term problems and personality difficulties. Schemas are very powerful, often self-defeating, negative beliefs (developed in childhood) about the way the world works. Examples include beliefs such as 'I am unlovable', 'People always leave me' and 'I can't trust anyone'. Although such beliefs are difficult to change, understanding them can help people to feel more in control when these beliefs are activated in stressful situations and in close relationships with others.

Essential guidelines (NICE guidelines on computerised CBT 2006)

There are five computer-based CBT programmes available. Two of these are recommended by NICE:

'Beating the blues' for depression
'Fear-fighter' for phobias

REFERENCES

NICE Clinical Guidelines (2006) *Computerised CBT*. National Institute for Clinical Excellence.
Timms, P. (ed) (2005). *Royal College of Psychiatrists Public Education Leaflet: Cognitive Behavioural Therapy*. RCPsych Public Education Editorial Board

COGNITIVE ANALYTIC THERAPY (CAT)

Description

'CAT is short for cognitive analytic therapy. In CAT the early sessions focus on the development of a shared understanding with the patient of their childhood experiences, and particularly on how any difficult experiences were dealt with and "survived". The emphasis is on how the person learnt to relate to others. These patterns of relating can become fixed or unhelpful and as the therapy progresses, the focus turns towards the recognition and revision of these unhelpful patterns in the present day.'

'It is cognitive because it uses the patient's capacity to observe and think about themselves, their assumptions, feelings and behaviour.'

'It is analytic in that recognition of early relationship patterns is central to the model, incorporating important aspects of object relations theory.'

How it works

CAT usually takes places over 16 weekly sessions with a follow-up three months after therapy ends. A longer CAT of 24 weeks is used for more complex cases.

In CAT the therapist and patient work closely together in a collaborative way. Use of the therapeutic relationship is central to the work of therapy.

CAT is usually used for individuals, but can also be used with couples, groups and in organisations.

Key terms

Procedures (or procedural sequences)

A procedure is a chain of mental processes and actions. Procedures include:

Snags

When the person sabotages success in their life either because of the fear of the response of others or because of something within themselves e.g. I must sabotage success (of the therapy) as I don't deserve it.

Traps

When a person's behaviour, based on a negative assumption, ends up confirming the negative assumption e.g. a person who feels worthless and anxious may try and please others, but may end up being taken advantage of which makes them angry, depressed or guilty, thereby confirming their original feelings.

Dilemmas

When a person believes that they can only act in one of two ways and each way is unsatisfactory e.g. a person who has been made to feel stupid in the past for talking about their feelings may feel that they have no other options than to bottle up their feelings or risk being ridiculed.

Psychotherapy file

Patients who engage in CAT are given a questionnaire in the first session, called the psychotherapy file. In this, patients identify common snags, traps and dilemmas which helps the therapist in the reformulation process.

Reformulation

The therapist writes a letter to the patient in the fourth or fifth session, which is a summary of the shared understanding he and the patient have reached so far. This includes a description of how events from the past have resulted in the patient developing patterns of relating that are no longer helpful. Target problem procedures are those traps, dilemmas and snags that have been identified to be worked on in therapy.

Recognition and revision
> A gradual process occurring over the remaining sessions after reformulation, whereby the patient learns to identify the unhelpful procedures and eventually find alternative strategies.

Reciprocal roles
> These are the roles learnt in childhood, usually derived from the relationship with both parents. So someone, for example, whose mother was very critical, is not only very familiar with the 'criticised' role, but also has learnt how to do the 'criticising' role. Both poles of this role become internalised at a level often beyond conscious awareness. These roles then are re-enacted in the person's relationships in the present day, including within the therapeutic relationship.

Goodbye letters
> These are written and read out in the final session by both the patient and the therapist. They usually provide a summary of the work done and identify any potential pitfalls anticipated once therapy ends.

REFERENCES

Association for Cognitive Analytic Therapy Online. www.acat.me.uk

Dryden, W. (ed.) (2007). *Dryden's Handbook of Individual Therapy* (5th edn). Sage pp. 287–96

Naismith, J. & Grant, S. (ed.).(2007) *College Seminars Series: Seminars in the Psychotherapies.* The Royal College of Psychiatrists (2007). pp. 118–139

DIALECTICAL BEHAVIOURAL THERAPY (DBT)

Description

'DBT is a type of talking therapy which was developed to help people who have problems controlling their emotions and who cope by harming themselves. It is often used for people with a borderline personality diagnosis or who self harm repeatedly.'

'During DBT people learn techniques to deal with painful emotions. By dealing with painful emotions, the patient can hope to address the self-destruction of self-harm.'

'It has links to cognitive behaviour therapy and to the theory of dialectics. Dialectic theory proposes that ideas and realities often have polarities or opposing aspects which need to be accepted.'

How it works

DBT can involve both individual and group work. DBT adherent therapy would include both.
At the outset, a therapy agreement is made which determines:
    attendance
    length of therapy
    circumstances which would lead to termination of therapy
    behaviours which are considered to be therapy interfering
    the need to attend skills training
    the obligation to resist suicidal behaviour
Prospective patients must demonstrate two or more of the following:
    emotional dysregulation e.g. anger problems
    interpersonal dysregulation e.g. unstable relationships
    behavioural dysregulation e.g. suicide threats
    cognitive dysregulation e.g. cognitive disturbances
    self dysfunction e.g. unstable self image

Key terms

Skills training (delivered in a group setting)
    (D) Distress tolerance skills
        Distress tolerance skills help to tolerate painful events and emotions when things cannot be made better right away
    (I) Interpersonal effectiveness skills
        Relationship effectiveness skills are geared at getting or keeping a good relationship
    (C) Core mindfulness
        Core mindfulness is a technique which enables you to be in control of your mind, instead of letting your mind be in control of you. It includes the idea of acceptance; i.e. by accepting that some suffering is inevitable in life for everyone, it can feel less awful when difficult situations do arise.
    (E) Emotion regulation
        Emotion regulation helps you to understand the emotions you experience and to identify what you can do to become less vulnerable to these emotions.
Telephone contact
    Telephone contact may be used to help the patient get through crises by using the skills learnt in the sessions. Telephone contact aims to reduce self harm during periods of crisis.

REFERENCES

Gelder, M., Harrison, P. & Cowen, P. (2001) *Shorter Oxford Textbook of Psychiatry* (5th edn) Oxford University Press p. 599

Linehan, M.M., Tutek, D.A., Heard, H.L. *et al.* (1994). Interpersonal outcome of cognitive behavioural treatment for chronically suicidal borderline patients. *American Journal of Psychiatry* **151**, 1777–6.

Palmer, R.L. (2002). Dialectical behaviour therapy for borderline personality disorder. *Advances in Psychiatric Treatment* **8**, 10–16

FAMILY THERAPY

Description

'Family therapy helps family members find constructive ways of helping each other. This is done by exploring each individual's perspectives and beliefs. Family therapy does not only help individuals change, it also improves family relationships and functioning.'

'Family therapy has been recommended in the government (NICE) guidelines as being helpful for several conditions such as schizophrenia, mood related conditions and eating disorders.'

How it works

Family therapy brings families together in sessions. Often all the family living at home would be invited initially and sometimes non family members or extended family members are included as well if they are involved in what is happening.

Family therapy helps to identify a family's strengths and weaknesses, e.g. an inability to confide in each other. It also helps to identify specific concerns and assesses how the family is handling them.

During family therapy the therapist will guide the family towards learning new ways of interacting and overcoming old problems.

Key terms

Structural family therapy

In this kind of therapy, the therapist helps the family to address problems within the family structure. For example, the therapist can help struggling parents to put proper boundaries in place for their children, and to assume a responsible, authoritative role within the family. Structural family therapy aims to restore hierarchies and challenge absent or rigid boundaries. In structural family therapy, the therapist may have to temporarily join with one member against another in order to achieve these aims. For example, if the therapist considers that the wife is particularly dependent on the husband, he may ask the wife what her husband does which makes her feel so dependent. Whilst this may cause tension in the short term, it is ultimately aimed at bringing about change.

Systemic family therapy

In systemic family therapy, the therapist often works in a team. One or two therapists will sit in the room with the family, while the team looks on from behind a one way mirror and helps to generate ideas and questions for the family to consider. This kind of therapy does not tend to focus on how problems within the family arose, nor who might be to 'blame', but instead looks at how the family is functioning now. The therapist helps the family to find their own solutions to difficulties by helping them to identify their strengths and the positive aspects of their relationships. Systemic family therapy is associated with circular questioning, in which one member of the family might be asked, for example to comment on the relationship between two other family members. This type of questioning can bring up new ideas and perspectives within the family that have not been heard before and encourages the family to recognise their own potential to see and do things differently. The therapist and team generate lots of ideas (hypotheses) about how the family system is functioning, which they can then test out with the family. The therapist then encourages the family to behave in different ways to help to resolve the conflicts which initially brought them to therapy.

REFERENCES

Asen, E. (2002) Outcome research in family therapy. *Advances in Psychiatric Treatment* **8**, 230–238

Gelder, M., Harrison, P. & Cowen, P. (2001) *Shorter Oxford Textbook of Psychiatry.* (5th edn) Oxford University Press. pp. 577–617

Naismith, J. & Grant, S. (ed.) (2007) *College Seminars Series: Seminars in the Psychotherapies.* The Royal College of Psychiatrists. pp. 235–260

The Association for Family Therapy. www.aft.org.uk

INDIVIDUAL PSYCHODYNAMIC PSYCHOTHERAPY

Description

'Psychodynamic psychotherapy is a kind of talking therapy which attempts to help people develop insight into deep seated problems that are usually thought to stem from childhood and significant relationships.'

'Psychodynamic psychotherapy was initially developed to help people with anxiety and phobias. However, this kind of therapy is now also used to help other people who have different problems such as interpersonal difficulties.'

'Psychodynamic therapy is also practised in groups. The groups have usually six to eight members plus one or two faciltiators (therapists). Group therapy grew out of a recognition that humans are fundamentally social, not solitary, animals, and that the way we relate to others in groups is important for our sense of well being. Groups use the same dynamic ideas as in individual therapy, but allow patients to explore both individual relationships and their relationship to the group as a whole.'

How it works

Traditionally therapy was given several times a week over several years. Whilst some people still attend therapy on this basis, others will need shorter courses of therapy.

Each session usually lasts for around 50 minutes, and usually takes place in the same place and at the same time. It is always with the same therapist.

Therapy is based on the relationship between the patient and the therapist.

There is less formal structure within the sessions than in other therapies such as CBT . For example during therapy, the patient is encouraged to speak about whatever comes to their mind. This is called free association.

The past may be talked about extensively in the therapy but the here and now and the relationship with the therapist in the room is also very important.

Key terms

Interpretation

A verbal intervention made by a therapist aimed at increasing insight. Often involves 'making the unconscious conscious' i.e. drawing attention to issues that have previously been out of the patient's awareness, so that these issues can be talked about and worked through.

Boundaries

This refers to the framework around the therapy; the regularity of time and place, and the way that the therapist ensures he relates to the patient in a professional, therapeutic and thoughtful way.

Transference

The unconscious redirection of feelings for one person to another. For example if a patient's father seemed to him to be cold and distant, he may also unwittingly come to see the therapist in a similar light, even if the therapist is in fact warm and interested. Exploring this can help the patient to understand more about how he views other people and can help him then to develop more healthy and fulfilling relationships with others.

Countertransference

The transfer of the therapist's own unconscious feelings to the patient or feelings generated within the therapist by the patient's unconscious.

Much of the way we communicate with others happens without words, and often even out of our awareness. One way we communicate with others is by arousing feelings in them (which is called countertransference when it happens in therapy). For example a person who is crying may elicit sympathy, while a person who is abrupt may make others feel rejected.

By tuning in to how patients make us feel during a therapy session, we can get very useful information about their relationships. For example, if a patient cannot express or acknowledge his angry feelings and so tends to be very passive, the therapist may find herself feeling angry or annoyed with the patient, he is picking up on the anger that the patient cannot feel. If he is picking this up, then it is likely that other people react to this patient in a similar way, and he can use this information to gently help the patient to explore his difficulties with anger, and to feel ok about expressing it more openly. In this example, it is important for the therapist to pay close attention to his own feelings too he may have his own reasons to be angry that day, and if he is not also tuned in to this, he may misinterpret what is happening with the patient.

Free association

Patients are asked to relate anything which comes into their minds, regardless of how superficially unimportant or potentially embarrassing the memory threatens to be.

Fantasy

Used to describe unconscious desires, fears, drives etc.

Resistance

Refers to the process whereby the patient (either directly or indirectly) opposes changing their behaviour, or refuses to discuss, remember, or think about clinically relevant experiences.

Psychotherapy contract

Sets out the rules for how the therapy will take place, e.g. how many sessions, how to resolve problems out of hours, what behaviours are acceptable and the rules for missed sessions and lateness.

Psychoanalysis

Psychoanalysis is a form of psychotherapy which is based on the psychoanalytic theories of psychoanalysts such as Freud, Winnicott and Klein. Psychoanalysis is concerned with exploring thoughts, fantasies, dreams and memories of childhood experiences. Whilst the practice of psychodynamic psychotherapy also developed out of psychoanalytic theory, there are important differences between the two therapies. Psychoanalysis usually takes place five times a week and will typically last a number of years, whereas the time-frame for psychodynamic psychotherapy is more flexible. In psychodynamic psychotherapy the therapist faces the patient thereby fostering a therapeutic relationship, whereas in psychoanalysis the patient usually reclines on a couch while the analyst faces *away* from them thereby adopting a blank slate onto which the patient will 'transfer' his feelings that they have towards important people in their life. Whilst the majority of psychoanalysis is funded privately by the patient, psychodynamic psychotherapy is available on the NHS.

Brief psychodynamic psychotherapy

As the name suggests, brief psychodynamic psychotherapy is limited to a brief series of sessions. The typical number of sessions is 10. Usually one theme is chosen jointly by the patient and the therapist, which becomes the focus of the therapy, e.g. bereavement or separation anxiety. The purpose of brief psychodynamic psychotherapy is to give the patient ways of understanding him/herself which can be generalised to other issues. It is not usually appropriate for people who have complex needs as seen in personality disorder.

REFERENCES

Gelder, M., Harrison, P. & Cowen, P. (2001) *Shorter Oxford Textbook of Psychiatry* (5th edn) Oxford University Press pp. 89–91 & 577–617

Naismith, J. & Grant, S. (eds) (2007) *College Seminars Series: Seminars in the Psychotherapies*. The Royal College of Psychiatrists pp. 100–117

COMPLEX NEEDS PROGRAMME

Description

'Complex needs is a term which is used for people with complicated lives, who have difficulties with relationships, and who are vulnerable to emotional and interpersonal problems. It had been recognised that existing services often did not fit the needs of such a complex group of clients.'
'Complex needs services were developed specifically to help these people, who often have personality disorders or recurrent self harm, and it can also help those with other diagnoses and those who have several diagnoses.'
'The programme provides patients with the opportunity to meet other people with similar difficulties on a regular basis and to work on issues together that they find particularly hard. Complex needs services often use a range of therapeutic approaches, often, but not always in groups. Many but not all services are based on a therapeutic community model. They often use the idea of involving users and recovered users in helping each other.'
'They often use clear contracts and boundaries around such key issues as recurrent self harm or addictive behaviour.'
'People with a personality disorder may benefit from the complex needs programme but other people may benefit too.'
'The services often offer long term help e.g. for 18 months or so and have various levels of therapy and attendance.'
'Some services discourage use of many therapeutic medications especially sedatives.'
'Often the services encourage self referral as well as other means of referral.'

Key terms

Therapeutic communities

A therapeutic community describes a group setting in which the members become the therapist for each other. By being part of the community the patient becomes more self aware and adapts his behaviour accordingly. Both therapists and patients form the community but in contrast to other sorts of psychotherapy, the patient and the therapist should not be immediately distinguishable. The users are often involved in the running of the community and a flat hierarchy is aimed for. The concept is based on many different therapeutic principles including analytic, behavioural, and cognitive. The experience of membership to a community fosters a greater understanding of social interaction and allows people to learn to take more responsibility for themselves. People with a range of problems (e.g. mental illness, substance misuse and offending behaviour) may benefit from being part of a therapeutic community.

REFERENCES

Association of Therapeutic Communities www.therapeuticcommunities.org
Keene, J. (2001) *Clients with complex needs.* Blackwell Publishing

Core information

There is no hard and fast rule when assessing someone's suitability for psychotherapy. However for the purposes of feeling confident in assessing or commenting on someone's suitability for psychotherapy as part of a CASC examination task, the following framework will help you demonstrate a sound working knowledge of the sorts of factors which should be considered.

Factors which suggest that the patient may be able to benefit from psychotherapy

Good ego strength

This means that the patient has a relatively stable sense of self, and can tolerate a certain amount of anxiety without feeling that they are falling apart. This can be tested by asking patients how they react in stressful situations e.g. do they use healthy strategies such as asking for support from loved ones, or do they react by harming themselves?

Psychological Mindedness

This describes an interest in the workings of one's own mind and how that might relate to how we behave with others.

An understanding of the proposed model of therapy

Put simply, if you like the sound of a particular kind of therapy, and feels it suits your way of thinking, then it is more likely to be effective for you.

Ability to form a therapeutic relationship

This is a key factor, as the research evidence suggests that the best predictor of a good outcome in therapy is the presence of a positive relationship between the therapist and patient. When assessing this, look for evidence that the patient has had at least one positive, trusting relationship in their lives (this may be with a previous therapist or counsellor, or may be with a loved one or friend).

Motivation

The patient's own motivation to change is a very powerful positive indicator that therapy will be helpful.

Factors which suggest that a patient may not be able to benefit from therapy

Actively psychotic or suicidal

Commencing therapy can be a stressful experience, as it involves learning new ways of dealing with things and challenging old and familiar patterns of behaviour. Ideally patients should be in a relatively stable, supported position when undertaking such work, so that they can derive the maximum benefit from it. If patients are actively psychotic, acutely suicidal, or their lives are extremely chaotic, they may need medication or practical support initially, and psychotherapy can again be considered when things have settled down.

Significant drug and alcohol use (including sedative medication)

If someone is taking mind altering substances as a means of controlling their distress, they will be less able to work on their emotions in therapy. Patients with significant difficulties in this area will need support to control their substance use before therapy begins. Practical techniques such as psychoeducation, supportive psychotherapy, motivational interviewing, or 12 step programmes such as Alcoholics Anonymous may be very helpful.

If you identify that someone has difficulties with any of the above examples, then psychotherapy may only be possible if the psychotherapeutic techniques can be modified. Otherwise, it may be appropriate to consider a completely different treatment approach.

REFERENCES

Gelder, M., Harrison, P. & Cowen, P. (2001) *Shorter Oxford Textbook of Psychiatry* (5th edn) Oxford University Press pp. 577–617

Naismith, J. & Grant, S. (ed) (2007) *College Seminars Series: Seminars in the Psychotherapies*. The Royal College of Psychiatrists pp. 1–27

Turkington, D., Dudley, R., Warman, D.M. *et al.* (2004). Cognitive-behavioural therapy for schizophrenia: a review. *Journal of Psychiatric Practice* **10**, 5–16

THE MENTAL HEALTH ACT (England and Wales)

Information giving

What is the Mental Health Act (MHA)?

'Sometimes mental illness can affect a person's ability to make decisions, or may cause them to act so that they hurt themselves, or rarely, other people. The Mental Health Act (1983) as amended in 2007 exists to ensure the safety, protection and treatment of people with mental illness.'

'We consider carefully whether the patient needs to be detained in the interests of the patient's own health or safety or with a view to the protection of other people.'

To whom does the Mental Health Act apply?

'The Mental Health Act can apply to anyone with a disorder or disability of mind'.

'Appropriate treatment must be available but need not be the most appropriate treatment or all the treatment. "Treatment" includes nursing, rehabilitation and care.'

Section 2

'We use Section 2 of the Act when we are of the opinion that a patient is suffering from a mental disorder of a nature or degree that warrants admission to hospital for an assessment. This can last for up to 28 days. This section cannot be renewed but can be converted to a Section 3.'

Section 3

'We use Section 3 of the Act to detain a person with a confirmed mental illness who needs in-patient treatment. This can last for up to six months. At the end of this period the section can be renewed for another six months. It can be renewed after this for periods of 12 months.'

Who does the section assessment?

'The section assessment is performed by two doctors, who make medical recommendations, and an Approved Mental Health Practitioner (AMHP), who makes the application. One of the doctors should be approved under Section 12(2) of the Act as having special experience in the diagnosis and treatment of mental disorder. The other doctor should have prior knowledge of the patient. Ideally one of the doctors is a psychiatrist and the other is the patient's GP.'

The appeal process

'The patient can appeal against the detention to the hospital managers or to the Mental Health Review Tribunal (MHRT). The MHRT consists of a legal representative, a consultant psychiatrist and a lay member. The tribunal can discharge a patient from a section, as can the Responsible Clinician (RC), the hospital managers and the nearest relative, unless the nearest relative is subject to a barring order.'

Treating physical illnesses

'Physical illnesses can only be treated when they give rise to psychiatric disorders, for example delirium, or when the psychiatric disorder leads to physical complications, as in eating disorders.

When a drug which requires regular blood monitoring, such as clozapine, is used for the treatment of a psychiatric disorder, then the necessary blood tests are allowed.'

Section 136

'The police can use Section 136 to bring a person suspected of being mentally ill to a place of safety.'

Section 17

'This section of the Act concerns periods of leave, which can only be authorised by the Responsible Clinician (RC), or by their deputy who has also been approved under the Act.'

Treatment under the Act

'Medication can be given for three months to patients subject to Section 3. After this time a Second Opinion Appointed Doctor (SOAD) must be asked to review the case.'

CAPACITY

Core information

Capacity is defined by Mental Capacity Act 2007 (England and Wales).

Assessing capacity

Explain the exact reason you are there
  Capacity for what?
Assessing capacity is everyone's responsibility
  Assume capacity unless shown otherwise
  An unwise decision does not mean lack of capacity
To have capacity an individual must be able to do all the following:
  Understand the information and retain it for long enough to reach a decision
  Use and weigh up the information to make a decision
  Communicate the decision
Lack of capacity
  Must be due to an impairment or disturbance of the functioning of the mind or the brain
  Can be permanent or temporary
Best interests
  Make all reasonable attempts to restore capacity or delay the decision until capacity is restored
  Consultant with everyone with whom it is reasonable
Advance decisions
  To refuse consent for health care or treatment in advance
  Can be verbal or written
  A 'do not resuscitate' order must be in writing
Lasting power of attorney
  Can now include decisions about health, as well as finances

Assessing testamentary capacity

Is aware what a will constitutes
  'What is a will?'
  'How would you go about making a will?'
  'What if your situation changes or you change your mind?'
Knows the general extent of their assets
  'What assets or belongings do you have to leave?'
  'How much are they worth?'
  'What about any savings and pension?'
Is aware of the people who might reasonably expect to benefit
  'Tell me about your family.'
  'What are their names?'
  'Who do you plan to leave your assets to?'
  'What claim do they have to your assets?'
Is free from delusional beliefs that may affect distribution
  Assess for delusional beliefs, as in psychosis
Not under the influence of any drugs that may distort mental capacity
  Alcohol, illicit drug and prescribed drug history
Brief screen for evidence of mental illness / cognitive impairment
Say whether you will come back and re-assess to assess consistency of thinking/decision

MENTAL HEALTH RESOURCES

Organisations

MIND	www.mind.org.uk
NHS Direct	www.nhsdirect.nhs.uk
Patient UK	www.patient.co.uk
SANE	www.sane.org.uk
The Royal College of Psychiatrists	www.rcpsych.ac.uk

Support groups and websites

Age Concern	www.ace.org.uk
Alcoholics Anonymous	www.alcoholics-anonymous.org.uk
Alzheimer's Society	www.alzheimers.org
Carers UK	www.carersuk.org
Childline	www.childline.org.uk
Contact a Family (children with LD)	www.cafamily.org.uk
CRUSE (bereavement)	www.crusebereavementcare.org.uk
Depression Alliance	www.depressionalliance.org
Mirror Mirror (eating disorders)	www.mirror-mirror.org
Motherisk (drugs in pregnancy)	www.motherisk.org
Narcotics Anonymous	www.ukna.org
National Autistic Society	www.nas.org
NHS Smoking Helpline	www.givingupsmoking.co.uk
OCD-UK	www.ocduk.org
Pendulum (bipolar disorder)	www.pendulum.org
Rethink (service provision)	www.rethink.org
Samaritans	www.samaritans.org.uk
Schizophrenia	www.schizophrenia.com
Self-harm Network	www.nshn.co.uk
Survivors UK (male rape victims)	www.survivorsuk.org
Talk to Frank (drug information)	www.talktofrank.com
The Gender Trust	www.gendertrust.org.uk
UK Council for Psychotherapy	www.psychotherapy.org.uk
YoungMinds (child mental health)	www.youngminds.org.uk

Books

Anger	Overcoming Irritability and Anger
Anorexia Nervosa	Overcoming Anorexia Nervosa
Anxiety	Overcoming Anxiety
Bulimia Nervosa	Overcoming Binge Eating
Depression	Overcoming Depression
Bipolar Disorder	Overcoming Mood Swings
Obsessive Compulsive Disorder	Overcoming OCD
Panic	Overcoming Panic
PTSD	Overcoming Traumatic Stress
Bereavement	You'll Get Over It: Rage of Bereavement
Stress	Managing Stress

COGNITIVE ASSESSMENT (MMSE)

Orientation

'What year is it?'	(1)
'What season are we in?'	(1)
'What month are we in?'	(1)
'What is today's date?'	(1)
'What day of the week is it?'	(1)
'What country are we in?	(1)
'What county are we in?'	(1)
'What town/city are we in?'	(1)
'What street are we on/ what building are we in?'	(1)
'What number building are we in/what floor are we on?'	(1)

Registration

'I'm going to name three objects. After I've finished saying them I want you to say them back to me. Then try to remember them and I will ask you them again later.
Say apple, table, penny, take a second to pronounce each word and repeat until all three are correct. (3)

Attention/concentration

'Please take seven away from 100, and then take seven from that number until I tell you to stop.' Or 'Spell WORLD backwards' (5)

Recall (after five minutes)

'Can you remember the three objects?' (apple, table, penny) (3)

Language/other

'Could you please name this object?' (pen/pencil, watch) (2)
Listen to this sentence and repeat after me 'No, ifs, ands or buts' (1)
Put a piece of paper on the desk and say 'Please take this piece of paper, fold it in half and put it on the floor.' (3)
'Please do what is written on this piece of paper' (Close your eyes) (1)
'Please write a complete sentence on this piece of paper. It can be anything you like and it doesn't have to be long' (1)
'Please copy this drawing as best you can, it does not have to be perfect' (Intersecting pentagons) (1)

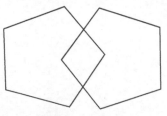

CLOSE YOUR EYES

Thank the patient.

Extras (not part of MMSE)

If there is time perform a clock face drawing test.
Some CASC stations may be combinations of cognitive tests e.g. MMSE and frontal lobe.

Abbreviated mental test (Hodkinson)

Patient's age	(1)
Time (to the nearest hour)	(1)
Address e.g. 42 West Street (to be recalled at end of test)	(1)
Year	(1)
Name of the hospital or number of the residence	(1)
Recognition of two people	(1)
Day and month of birth	(1)
Date of World War I	(1)
Name of monarch or prime minister	(1)
Count backwards from 20 down to one	(1)

REFERENCES

Folstein, M.F., Folstein, S.E. & McHugh, P.R. (1975) Mini-Mental State: A practical method for grading the cognitive state of patients for the clinician. *Journal of Psychiatric Research*, **12**, 189–198

Hodkinson, H.M. (1972) Evaluation of a mental test score for assessment of mental impairment in the elderly. *Age and Ageing*, **1**(4) 233–238

ASSESSING FRONTAL LOBE FUNCTION

The following tests provide a structured approach to assessing frontal lobe function. You may find that you do not have enough time to perform every test.

Personality

'Have you changed in yourself in any way?'

'Do other people ever say you have changed?'

'In what way?'

Verbal fluency

Letter fluency

'I would like you to come up with as many words as you can think of beginning with the letter S in one minute. Try and make all the words different and try not to use names.'

Category fluency

'I would like you to tell me the names of as many animals as you can think of in one minute.'

Abstraction

Proverb interpretation

'I would like you to tell me what you understand by the following phrases'

'Too many cooks spoil the broth'

'One swallow doesn't make a summer'

Cognitive estimates

'I would like you to make the best guess you can in answer to these questions'

'How tall is the average English woman?'

'What is the best-paid job in Britain today?'

Abstract similarities

'I would like you to tell me how the following items are similar:

'apple and banana'

'poem and statue'

Response-inhibition and set-shifting

Motor sequencing (Luria's test)

'I would like you watch my hand movements'

Demonstrate the hand sequence (fist-edge-palm) five times without giving verbal clues

'Now I would like you to copy those movements'

Go/No Go

'When I touch my nose, you raise your finger like this'

'When I raise my finger, you touch your nose like this'

Executive functioning

Key finding task

Draw a box on a piece of paper and show the drawing to the patient.

'I would like you to imagine that this box is a field. Now I would like you to imagine that earlier today you went for a walk in this field. However when you got home you realised that you must have lost a key in the field. I would now like you to show me how you would go about finding the key by tracing the path you would take with this pen.'

REFERENCES

Hodges, J.R. (1994) *Cognitive Assessment for Clinicians.* Oxford University Press pp. 108–154

ASSESSING PARIETAL LOBE FUNCTION

The following tests provide a structured approach to assessing parietal lobe function. You may find that you do not have enough time to perform every test.

Dominant parietal lobe function
Receptive dysphasia (obvious from conversation)
Screening for Gerstmann's syndrome
  Finger agnosia:
  'Point your right index finger at me'
  Dyscalculia:
  'What does 4 + 7 equal?'
  Right—left orientation:
  'Show me your left hand'
  Agraphia:
  'I would like you to write a couple of sentences for me'

Non-dominant parietal lobe function
Neglect (inattention)
  'I would like you draw a clock face, put in the numbers and show me the time so it shows five to the hour'
Anosagnosia (if you are told the patient has an impairment)
  Ask patient about their physical impairment
Constructional apraxia
  'I would like you to copy these drawings'
  Draw a cube and two intersecting pentagons as found in the figure in section *Cognitive assessment (MMSE)*
Topographical disorientation
  'Do you ever find yourself getting confused or lost in new places?'

Bilateral lobe function
Astereognosia
  'I would like you to close your eyes, I am then going to place an object in the palm of your hand and I would like you to tell me what it is without looking at it'
  Place a key/coin into the palm of the patient's hand.
Agraphagnosia
  'Once again I would like you to close your eyes. This time I am going to trace a letter onto the palm of your hand and I would like you to tell me which letter it is'
  Trace either an H or a W onto the palm of the patient's hand.

For completion
Assess visual fields to elicit lower homonymous quadrantanopia
Prosopagnosia
  Explain that prosopagnosia is a recognised deficit seen in patients with both parietal and temporal lobe impairment. Mention that this deficit may be elicited using an instrument such as the Benton Facial Recognition Test.

REFERENCES
Hodges, J.R. (1994) *Cognitive Assessment for Clinicians*. Oxford University Press pp. 108–154

ASSESSING TEMPORAL LOBE FUNCTION

The following tests provide a structured approach to assessing temporal lobe function. You may find that you do not have enough time to perform every test.

Dominant lobe
Receptive dysphasia
> This should be obvious from the conversation.

Alexia
> 'I would like you to read a couple of sentences from this page please'
> Give the patient something to read. (This could be a copy of the instructions you were given for the CASC station.)

Agraphia
> 'Now I would like you to write a couple of sentences for me'

Impaired learning and retention of verbal material
> 'I am going to give you a name and an address and I would like you to repeat it: John Green, 42 West Register Street, Luton, Bedfordshire'
> Ask patient to recall it three to five minutes later after interposing other cognitive tests.

Non-dominant lobe
Visuospatial difficulties

Anomia
> 'I am now going to point at a few items and I would like you to give me their names'
> Show patient a series of objects whose names are of increasing difficulty, e.g. pen, watch, nib and buckle.

Hemisomatopagnosia (e.g. if you are told patient is hemiplegic)
> 'Are all four of your limbs healthy and working well?'
> A patient with hemisomatopagnosia would tell you he is missing one side of his body.

Impaired learning and retention on non-verbal material
> 'I would like you to copy this drawing I am making up'
> It is important to draw something abstract because you will need to ask the patient to copy it from memory in five minutes and a picture of a cat, for example, will be easily remembered.

Bilateral
Assessing memory
> Short-term
> 'What did you eat for breakfast?'
> 'How did you get here today?'
> Famous events
> 'What happened to JF Kennedy?'
> 'Can you tell me why the twin towers fell in New York?'
> Remote personal (autobiographical):
> 'Where were you born?'
> 'Can you describe your first day at school?'

For completion
Assess visual fields to elicit upper homonymous quadrantanopia

Epileptic phenomena
> 'Have you ever had a fit?'
> 'Have you ever lost consciousness?'

Psychosis
> 'Has anything strange or unaccountable ever happened to you?'
> 'Have you ever heard voices when no one else is around?'

Prosopagnosia

Explain that prosopagnosia is a recognised deficit seen in patients with both parietal and temporal lobe impairment. Mention that this deficit may be elicited using an instrument such as the Benton Facial Recognition Test.

REFERENCES

Hodges, J.R. (1994) *Cognitive Assessment for Clinicians.* Oxford University Press pp. 108–154

Lishman, W.A. (1998) *Organic Psychiatry: The Psychological Consequences of Cerebral Disorder* (3rd edn) Blackwell Science pp. 94–148

CARDIOVASCULAR EXAMINATION

Introduction
> Introduce yourself
> Ask permission
> Ask if patient has pain anywhere
> Ask patient to inform you if you cause them any discomfort
> Ask them to expose their upper body
> Position patient at 45 degrees

The examination
> Inspect hands (temperature, pallor, clubbing, cyanosis, and vasculitis)
> Palpate radial and brachial pulses (rate, rhythm, synchronisation, water-hammer)
> Inspect extensor surface of elbow for xanthoma
> Palpate carotid pulses (character), listen for bruits
> Assess jugular venous pressure (JVP), measure height above sternal angle (normal = < 3cm)
> Inspect eyes (anaemia, xanthelasma, corneal arcus)
> Make a show of looking for malar rash
> Inspect mouth and tongue (central cyanosis, high arched palate of Marfan's)
> Inspect for scars, palpate over precordium for location, heaves and character of apex beat
> Palpate over four areas for thrills
> Auscultate in four valve areas for heart sounds, murmurs, added sounds (feel carotid pulse at the same time)
>> Aortic stenosis (listen for radiation to carotids)
>> Aortic regurgitation (sit patient forward, listen in held expiration at left sternal edge)
>> Tricuspid regurgitation (listen in held inspiration, feel for hepatic engorgement)
>> Mitral regurgitation (listen for radiation to axilla)
>> Mitral stenosis (turn patient on left, use bell, listen in held expiration at the apex)
> Palpate femoral pulses, check for radio-femoral delay
> Palpate peripheral pulses, popliteal, posterior tibial, dorsalis pedis, ankle oedema
> Auscultate lung bases for pulmonary oedema, breath sounds, sacral oedema
> Auscultate over femorals and abdominal aorta for bruits, look for ascites

For completion
> Ask for blood pressure/take blood pressure
> Explain that you would usually consider investigations such as an electrocardiogram, chest X-ray, blood tests, and an echocardiogram.

REFERENCES
Douglas, G., Nicol, F. & Robertson, C. (2005) *Macleod's Clinical Examination* (11th edn) Churchill Livingstone

RESPIRATORY EXAMINATION

Introduction
Introduce yourself
Ask permission
Ask if patient has pain anywhere
Ask patient to inform you if you cause them any discomfort
Ask them to expose their upper body
Position patient at 45 degrees

The examination
Examine the patient's hands (warmth, cyanosis, clubbing, tar staining)
Ask patient to hold hands out in front with wrists fully extended to observe for CO_2 flap
Feel for the radial pulse for 15 seconds and then without changing your position look at the patient's chest to measure their respiratory rate for 30 seconds
Examine the eyes for anaemia
Examine the mouth for central cyanosis (look under the tongue)
Examine JVP
Examine the chest anteriorly
Inspection
Shape of chest, scars, respiratory movements
Palpation
Trachea, chest expansion, tactile vocal fremitus ('say 99' and feel with ulnar edge of hand or ball of hand)
Percussion
Percuss over the clavicles and then several areas on each side, compare right with left
Auscultation
Auscultate in several areas on each side, compare right with left
Repeat for posterior chest

For completion
Ask for blood pressure/take blood pressure
Explain that you would usually consider investigations such as a chest X-ray, peak flow, blood tests, blood gases as well as the inspection of a sputum sample.

REFERENCES
Douglas, G., Nicol, F. & Robertson, C. (2005) *Macleod's Clinical Examination* (11th edn) Churchill Livingstone

ABDOMINAL EXAMINATION

For alcohol related signs see *Substance misuse* section.

Introduction

Introduce yourself

Ask permission

Ask if patient has pain anywhere

Ask patient to inform you if you cause them any discomfort

Ask them to expose abdomen (it will not be appropriate to request exposure of genitals)

Position patient lying supine with their hands by their sides

The examination

Inspect the hands

Clubbing, Dupuytren's contracture, palmar erythema

Inspect the abdomen

Obvious masses, scars, jaundice, abdominal distension, spider naevi, ascites, venous distension (caput medusae)

Ask patient to cough to inspect for hernias

Inspect chest for gynecomastia

Palpation

All nine areas, light then deep

Assess for rigidity, guarding, tenderness and rebound tenderness

Percussion

All nine areas

Right iliac region to right hypochondriac region for liver

Right iliac region to left hypochondriac for spleen

Auscultation

All four quadrants for bowel sounds

For completion

Explain that you would ideally perform a rectal and pelvic examination. Mention that you would inspect for specific signs such as testicular atrophy.

Explain that you would usually consider investigations such as an abdominal X-ray and blood tests.

REFERENCES

Douglas, G., Nicol, F. & Robertson, C. (2005) *Macleod's Clinical Examination* (11th edn) Churchill Livingstone

NEUROLOGICAL EXAMINATION

For cranial nerve examination see earlier.

Introduction

Introduce yourself

Ask permission

Ask if patient has pain anywhere

Ask patient to inform you if you cause them any discomfort

The examination

Inspection

Standing

Walking

At 45 degrees

Tone

Ask patient to relax

Extend each joint slowly at first and then more rapidly

Upper limb

Shoulder, elbow and wrist

Lower limb

Internal/external rotation and knee lift

Ankle clonus

Power

Upper limb

Shoulder shrug against resistance

Abduct (lateral direction) shoulders against resistance

Flex elbows against resistance

Extend wrists against resistance

Abduct fingers against resistance

Lower limb

Flex knees against resistance

Plantar flexion against resistance

Toe extension against resistance

Hip abduction against resistance

Reflexes

Upper limb

biceps, supinator and triceps

Lower limb

knee jerk, ankle jerk, plantar

Sensation

Proprioception

Eyes closed, start distal move proximal until impairment goes

Vibration sense

128 Hz tuning fork, test first on sternum, start distal move proximal

Pin-prick

Test first on sternum, move around systematically

Temperature

Use cold object and assess for quality

Light touch

Use cotton wool and assess for quality

Two point discrimination

Eyes closed, use opened out paperclip, apply either one or two ends, and ask them to state how many. Then determine the minimum distance at which two pints can be perceived.

Coordination

Finger-nose test

Rapid alternating movement of hands

Heel-shin test

Heel-toe gait

For completion

Explain that you would usually consider investigations such as an electroencephalogram (EEG), lumbar puncture and blood tests.

REFERENCES

Douglas, G., Nicol, F. & Robertson, C. (2005) *Macleod's Clinical Examination* (11th edn) Churchill Livingstone

CRANIAL NERVE EXAMINATION

Introduction
　Introduce yourself
　Ask permission
　Ask if patient has pain anywhere
　Ask patient to inform you if you cause them any discomfort
The examination
CNI (Olfactory)
If test substances are available check nasal passages are clear, test each nostril separately, by occluding opposite nostril, ask patient to identify each smell.
CNII (Optic)
Visual acuity (Snellen chart)
Pupillary reflexes
　Direct and consensual reflex
　use pen torch (with patient looking into distance to avoid accommodation response).
　Accomodation reflex
　ask patient to look at distant object then close-by object to assess pupil change.
Visual fields, colour vision (Ishihara plates), fundoscopy
CNs III, IV and VI (Oculomotor, Trochlear & Abducens)
Eye movements; use an 'H' shape.
CN V (Trigeminal)
Sensory
　Light touch and pain sensation in all three divisions, comparing left to right.
Motor
　Inspect for muscle wasting.
　Palpate masseters whilst patient clenches teeth.
　Reflexes (jaw-jerk)
CN VII (Facial)
Inspect for asymmetry
Motor
　Raise eyebrows
　Close eyes against resistance
　Bare teeth, blow out against closed mouth.
Taste (ideally would test taste with test substances)
CN VIII (Vestibulocochlear)
Hearing
　Test by rubbing fingers on one side and ask patient to repeat whispered words from the other. Consider Rinne's and Weber's tests if time and equipment permits.
Nystagmus (induce positional nystagmus using Hallpike's test)
Oculocephalic reflex (brisk passive rotation of head induces nystagmus)
CN IX and X (Glossopharyngeal and Vagus)
Observe movements of palate and uvula by asking patient to say 'aah.'
Ask patient to speak to assess whether it is hoarse or nasal.
Ask patient to cough to assess whether it is bovine or nasal.
CN XI (Accessory)
Inspect trapezius; ask patient to shrug shoulders, and against resistance
Inspect sternomastoids; ask patient to turn head against resistance
CN XII (Hypoglossal)
Ask patient to protrude tongue, and then waggle it from side to side
Ask patient to push tongue against inside of cheek and palpate
Ask patient to say 'lah lah lah' as quickly as possible

For completion

Explain that whilst a full examination of the cranial nerves would include testing of the corneal and gag reflexes, they are unpleasant and are therefore inappropriate for an examination setting.

If equipment (e.g. tuning fork) or test substances (e.g. for smell) have not been provided, acknowledge this to demonstrate a comprehensive knowledge of cranial nerve examination.

REFERENCES

Douglas, G., Nicol, F. & Robertson, C. (2005) *Macleod's Clinical Examination* (11th edn) Churchill Livingstone

OPHTHALMOSCOPY

Introduction
Introduce yourself
Ask permission
Ask if patient has pain anywhere
Ask patient to inform you if you cause them any discomfort
Explain procedure

The examination
Ask the patient to look at a distant object and blink and breathe normally.
Stand or sit on the side to be examined, an arm's length from the patient, and with your eyes level with the patient's eyes.
The ophthalmoscope should be set on the '0' lens.
To look at the right eye, hold the ophthalmoscope in the right hand.
Use the right eye to examine the patient's right eye (and use the left eye whilst examining the patient's left eye).
Switch on the instrument and shine it at the pupil, angling it slightly towards the nose.
If the eye closes, open it gently.
Demonstrate the red reflex and note the nature of any opacities in the media, which will be outlined black against the glow.
Keeping the beam pointing in the same, slightly nasal, direction and with the red reflex in view, move close to the patient, stopping just clear of the lashes.
Steady the instrument by resting the middle and ring fingers of the right hand against the patient's cheek.
The optic nerve (disc) should now be in view because of the angle of approach. If, instead of the disc, retinal blood vessels are seen, the 'arrow' made at bifurcations, points to the disc.
If the image is out of focus, use the index finger of the right hand to rotate the lens wheel until the view is clear.
Examine the fundus systematically.
Note any abnormality as though the fundus were a clock with the disc in its centre. The disc diameter (1.5mm) is used as the unit of measurement, e.g. 'I can see a haemorrhage at six o'clock, two disc diameters from the disc.'
Examine the macula last (although it is difficult to see through an undilated pupil). Use a narrow beam and ask the patient to look straight at the light. Look for the pigmentary changes of age-related macular degeneration and the exudates of diabetic maculopathy.

For completion
Mention that under ideal circumstances, you would use a dark room
Explain that it is usually necessary to dilate the pupil with an agent like tropicamide 1% in order to get a good view of the retina.

Findings in papilloedema
Swollen disc, congested veins, surrounding small haemorrhages, blurred disc margins, loss of cup.

Findings in diabetic retinopathy
Early
Dot and blot haemorrhages and microaneurysms
Late
Retinal ischaemia (cotton wool spots), venous dilatation and intra-retinal new vessels

Findings in proliferative retinopathy
Neovascularization sprouting from the optic nerve and retinal surface

REFERENCES
Douglas, G., Nicol, F. & Robertson, C. (2005) *Macleod's Clinical Examination* (11th edn) Churchill Livingstone
Khaw, P.T. & Elkington, A.R. (1999) *ABC of Eyes* (3rd edn) BMJ Books

ECG INTERPRETATION

One small square = 0.04 seconds
Five small squares = 1 big square = 0.2 seconds
Rate
  Divide 300 by the number of large squares between each QRS complex.
Rhythm
  Regular vs. irregular. Lay a piece of paper alongside the ECG and mark the position of three
  successive R waves. Check if the intervals are the same.
Axis
  Normal axis is between −30° and +90°. If the QRS complexes in leads I and II are
  predominantly positive then the axis is normal. Left axis deviation if lead I is positive but leads
  II and avF are negative. Right axis deviation if lead I is negative and leads II and avF are
  positive.
P waves
  Normal height (<2.5mm) and width (<0.11sec) are less than three small squares
  (3mm or 0.12 sec)
PR interval
  0.12–0.20 sec (three to five small squares)
QRS complex
  <0.12 sec (three small squares)
Q waves
  Pathological if more than 25% of the height of the following R wave or more than 0.04 sec
  (one small square) wide
ST segment
  Elevation suggests myocardial infarction or pericarditis
  Depression suggests myocardial ischaemia or left ventricular hypertrophy
T waves
  Inversion in leads I, II or V4–V6 is usually abnormal
  Peaked in hyperkalaemia, flattened in hypokalaemia
QT interval
  Between the beginning of the QRS complex and the end of the T wave
  QT must be corrected to QTc (corrected for heart rate)
  Given in milliseconds should be <440ms for men, <470ms for women
  Evidence suggests <500ms is ok (Maudsley 9th edition)
  As a rough guide at normal heart rate QT<2 big squares is ok (420ms)
Remember
  Tricyclics can provoke arrhythmias (prolong QRS interval)
  SSRIs can interact with warfarin but safe for QTc
  Some antipsychotics can prolong QTc
    Worst offenders are haloperidol, chlorpromazine and quetiapine
In a suspected myocardial infarction or myocardial ischaemia:
  Full history
  Full examination
  Contact the medical registrar
  Give oxygen and attach to a cardiac monitor if possible

REFERENCES
Hampton, J. The ECG Made Easy (7th edn) (2008) Churchill Livingstone
Taylor, D., Paton, C. & Kerwin, R. (2007) The Maudsley Prescribing Guidelines (9th edn) Informa Healthcare

RESUSCITATION

Call for help
> The most important thing is to get a defibrillator on the scene as soon as possible.

Check the environment for dangers
> Ensure safety of yourself, bystanders and patient

Check responsiveness
> Shake and shout

Open airway
> Turn onto back
>
> Head tilt
>
> Chin lift (or jaw thrust if cervical spine injury suspected)
>
> Remove any visible obstructions

Check breathing
> Look, listen and feel, for no more than 10 seconds
>
> (optional to check for carotid pulse simultaneously)

If breathing normally put into recovery position

If not breathing and help has not arrived, leave the patient to go and get help

Perform chest compressions
> Hand in the middle of the chest
>
> Depress 4–5 cm
>
> Compression and release take equal time
>
> Do not remove your hands from the sternum
>
> Deliver 30 compressions at a rate of 100 per minute

Deliver two effective rescue breaths
> Re-open airway
>
> Close nostrils
>
> Make good seal around mouth
>
> One second to inflate chest
>
> Observe chest falling
>
> Take a breath for yourself

Continue at rate of 30:2

State if another rescuer was present you would take over CPR from each other every two minutes. Do not stop to re-check patient.

Stop only if
> Normal breathing resumes.
>
> You are too exhausted to continue.
>
> Help arrives and takes over.

REFERENCES

Resuscitation Guidelines (2005) Resuscitation Council (UK)

MOCK EXAMINATIONS

HOW TO USE THE MOCK EXAMINATIONS

This section contains ten mock examinations. Each mock, as in the CASC examination itself, includes eight individual stations and four paired stations. This gives a total of 160 stations for you to choose from. It would probably take too long to go through a whole mock examination in one sitting. However gathering the stations together in this way will give you a general picture of the CASC examination.

We suggest that this book is used by study groups so that candidates can practise performing under examination conditions. Ideally the group should have at least three people, so that one person can act as the candidate, another take the role of the actor and the other plays the examiner.

If you can, arrange to meet in a room where you will not be disturbed. You could record the stations using a dictation machine or even a video camera. Your hospital's education centre may have such equipment.

Recording yourself may be nerve-racking, but it will help prepare you for the anxiety of the proper examination. It will also show you how you sound to others, and may highlight any overused phrases. One potential pitfall is the use of 'OK'; it is rarely appropriate to say this as you will mostly be listening to distressing histories and the use of 'OK' gives the impression that you are trivializing the patient's experiences.

Video recording has the added benefit of showing you how you appear to others, and may reveal problem areas such as unsatisfactory body language. This is important because body language may affect your overall score in a given station.

You will notice that there are several stations on key topics such as psychosis and depression. You cannot afford to be ill-prepared for these common topics. You will also notice that most mocks contain some difficult stations from the sub-specialties. It is unusual for the College to include more than a couple of problem stations in any one examination sitting, so you may wonder whether they are worth practising. However, whilst such stations are often included to differentiate high-achieving candidates, they are nonetheless important to prepare, as you will feel more confident that you have covered enough material. Having to talk about something you know little about will make you feel anxious and could affect your performance in other stations.

Possible areas of concern for all stations:

1. Questioning style e.g. use of appropriate mix of open and closed questions

2. Listening and responding appropriately to interviewee/discussant

3. Management of interview/examination including empathic responses

4. Appropriate focus for the required task

5. Fluency of interview/examination/discussion

6. Professionalism

Suggested points to cover:

For each mock examination station we have included at least three suggested main areas to cover. These points are not intended to be all inclusive but rather are suggestions on the sorts of areas that may be covered by more able candidates. We hope that these points will stimulate thought and discussion about where different scenarios may take the candidate. We feel that there are a wide variety of possible areas to cover and in the CASC exam your response will vary according to the specific instructions outside the booth and the actor found inside. Candidates are not rewarded for a pre-rehearsed script-like response. The CASC exam is about the flexible and responsive application of skills and knowledge.

MOCK EXAMINATION 1

Paired stations

1A You are working with the liaison team. You have been asked to go and see a 57-year-old woman who went to A&E with abdominal pain and soon vomited a large volume of fresh blood. She is haemodynamically stable and the medical registrar wants to perform endoscopy to treat her. However she is refusing to undergo the procedure. The registrar is concerned about the amount of blood loss, and has asked you to assess her capacity.

Suggested points to cover:

1. Does she understand and retain the information given?

2. Can she weigh up the information?

3. Can she communicate her decision?

1B Following your assessment you have been asked to report back to your consultant to discuss your findings. You believe that the patient lacks capacity to refuse endoscopy. You have told the patient this and she has become extremely distressed and has accused you of wanting to assault her.

Suggested points to cover:

1. Explain the reasoning that she lacks capacity.

2. Explain what you think the cause is.

3. Consider ways to restore capacity.

2A You have been asked to see Cerys, a 22-year-old secretary who has been feeling low in mood for several weeks. She told her GP she does not look forward to things anymore and has been finding it difficult to concentrate on her work. The GP believes she has mild depression and has asked you to discuss CBT with her. You should speak to the patient, making sure you address her fears and expectations.

Suggested points to cover:

1. Acknowledge patient's experience of depression.

2. Explain how talking therapy is known to help with symptoms of depression.

3. Explain what cognitive behavioural therapy involves.

2B You are now about to see the patient's mother, who is annoyed that you have not given her daughter any medication. She is demanding that you prescribe her an antidepressant as she knows that talking will not help. You should address the mother's fears and concerns. You should assume that the patient has given you her consent to talk to her mother.

Suggested points to cover:

1. Allow mother time to express her frustration.

2. Acknowledge her frustration.

3. Explain that clinical experience has shown that people with mild depression benefit most from psychological treatments like CBT.

3A You have been asked to see a 25-year-old man who has presented to A&E with chest pain. Physical examination and ECG were both normal. The patient was not happy with the assessment and became terrified when he was told he could go. He said that both his father and uncle have angina. In the past he was seen by a consultant cardiologist in the hospital, who concluded that the pain sounded like panic. Take a history from the patient and explain to him that his problems seem to be mainly psychological.

Suggested points to cover:

1. Take a history of pain symptoms.
2. Enquire about anxiety symptoms.
3. Explain how anxiety can cause these symptoms.

3B After you saw the patient, his mother approached you by the nurses' station to ask if you could meet with her to discuss her son. You should assume that the patient has given you his consent for you to do this. You take his mother to an interview room where she becomes very upset. She said that he is so concerned about his heart that he will only eat fish and rice and is too scared to go to work. She wants to know what is happening to him. You should explain his symptoms in a way she can understand and discuss ways in which you may be able to help them both.

Suggested points to cover:

1. Explain how anxiety can cause these symptoms and address concerns.
2. Discuss role of medication.
3. Discuss other treatment options e.g. CBT.

4A You have been asked to assess a 27-year-old man who is in police custody. He was arrested after police were called to a shopping mall where he was observed stealing a games console from an electrical store. He was recorded on CCTV. The custody sergeant was concerned about his 'mental ability' and interviewed him with an appropriate adult. The man has a mild learning disability. You should meet him to assess whether he is fit to plead in Magistrates' court.

Suggested points to cover:

1. Does he understand the nature of the charge?
2. Does he understand the difference between pleading guilty and not guilty?
3. Does he understand what will happen in court?

4B You are about to see the consultant to discuss the case. She knows the patient and informs you that he has a history of shoplifting and that six years ago he tried to take a handbag from an old lady. You should inform the consultant whether you consider that the patient is fit to plead. You will also be expected to discuss further management options.

Suggested points to cover:

1. Explain evidence behind your decision about fitness to plead.
2. Discuss his risk of re-offending.
3. Discuss the role of mental health services.

Individual stations

1 You have been asked to see a 36-year-old man in your outpatient clinic. Six weeks ago there was a fire at his home. He had to rescue his 18-month-old baby from an upstairs bedroom. Both of them survived, but the baby sustained serious burns and the patient is now complaining of problems sleeping and difficulties concentrating. Take a history paying particular attention to the problems since the fire.

Suggested points to cover:

1. Discuss the circumstances around the fire.

2. Elicit symptoms of PTSD.

3. Consider future risk to the baby and suicide risk.

2 You have been asked to see a patient in police custody. He has been charged with arson. The police surgeon said that the patient has been laughing to himself, and that he has refused to eat the meal he was given claiming that it was contaminated. Examine his mental state and elicit signs of psychosis.

Suggested points to cover:

1. Enquire about food and other possible delusions.

2. Enquire about auditory hallucinations.

3. Consider level of insight.

3 A 20-year-old lady is in A&E having taken six tablets of diazepam 2mg. Take a history and do a risk assessment with a view to admission or discharge. The nurses are concerned that this is her third overdose in two weeks and want her admitted.

Suggested points to cover:

1. Discuss the circumstances around the overdose.

2. Ascertain level of impulsivity.

3. Enquire about perceived consequences.

4 You have been asked to see the mother of a 7-year-old boy who you has just been diagnosed with autism. She is worried that it is her fault for allowing him to have the MMR vaccination. She tells you that she did not believe the link between the MMR vaccination and autism at the time, but now she cannot help feeling guilty. She wants to know more about the condition and what she should expect in the future.

Suggested points to cover:

1. Explain the basis of the difficulties in autism.

2. Explain no proven link with MMR vaccine.

3. Explain prognosis.

5 An 83-year-old lady is brought to A&E to see you. She has been picked up by the police wandering in the town centre at 3am. Assess her cognitive functioning.

Suggested points to cover:

1. Perform MMSE.

2. Ask what she was doing in the town centre at 3am.

3. Explore insight.

6 A 56-year-old grandmother has presented to A&E to request that her seven-year-old grandson is examined by a doctor to prove that he is the messiah. The A&E officer has told you that the woman

is 'talking nonsense' and that he is concerned about the safety of the patient's grandson after the patient said he can walk on water. You should assess the woman to elicit signs of psychosis, and to make an assessment of her risk.

Suggested points to cover:

1. Discuss her beliefs about the grandson.

2. Ask what she will do about this.

3. Enquire about other psychotic phenomenon.

7 You are working in substance misuse. You have been referred a 36-year-old man who is dependent on heroin. His partner has just died from a heroin overdose and he wishes to give up his own addiction. He has come to see you to discuss management options. He also wants to find out about HIV testing as he has recently watched a documentary on the risks of drug addiction. You do not need to confirm dependence.

Suggested points to cover:

1. Enquire what he already knows.

2. Explain how opiate detoxification works.

3. Offer HIV testing counselling and discuss harm minimization.

8 A 40-year-old man with a diagnosis of schizophrenia has come to your outpatient clinic. You notice that he has a resting tremor and that he is making bizarre chewing movements. You are concerned that he has developed extra-pyramidal side effects from his medication. He is currently receiving a depot antipsychotic medication every fortnight (flupentixol). You should examine him to elicit the signs of extra-pyramidal side effects. You should not attempt a full neurological examination.

Suggested points to cover:

1. Ask about what difficulties these movements produce.

2. Enquire about his attitude to his medication.

3. Discuss previous medication and future options.

MOCK EXAMINATION 2

Paired stations

1A You are about to see Sally Brown. She has been using heroin for two years and is concerned she may be pregnant. She has been seen in the drug and alcohol clinic over the last three months with a view to starting replacement therapy. She has a history of sharing needles and a history of unprotected sex. She wants to give up heroin. Address her concerns.

Suggested points to cover:

1. Explain possible risks of continued use of street heroin in pregnancy.
2. Explain possible risks of opiate replacement programmes in pregnancy.
3. Discuss harm minimization.

1B You receive a call from her GP. She is now confirmed as pregnant. Although the patient had a community detoxification soon after she saw you, the GP suspects that she may be injecting heroin again. You should talk to the GP to offer management advice. You should also discuss the potential risks to the unborn child.

Suggested points to cover:

1. Explain the importance of replacement therapy to reduce risks.
2. Discuss possible options for detoxification.
3. Suggest agencies for further help and advice.

2A You are asked to talk to Mohammed who is 20. He is complaining of pain in the back of his head. All investigations, including a CT scan have revealed nothing. His uncle had cancer and he is worried that he might have it now. Take a history of the pain and associated symptoms. Do not discuss diagnosis or management.

Suggested points to cover:

1. Take a history of the pain symptoms.
2. What do these symptoms mean to him?
3. Exclude depression.

2B His girlfriend wants to know what is wrong with him. Talk to her to explain the probable diagnosis and management and address any concerns she has.

Suggested points to cover:

1. Explain probable psychological cause e.g. tension headache.
2. Explain the headaches are not harmful.
3. Explain possible treatments e.g. relaxation.

3A You have been asked to see an 83-year-old woman who has been admitted to the medical ward from a local nursing home. The manager of the nursing home said that the woman has been hostile to the nursing staff and has been convinced that people have been taking things from her room. She also believes that people are purposefully moving her ornaments around. You should perform a mental state examination to elicit psychotic symptoms. You should also briefly assess her cognition.

Suggested points to cover:

1. Clarify whether she has ideas of persecution.

2. Assess orientation in time, place and person.

3. Assess mood.

3B The patient's daughter has just arrived on the ward. She wants to talk to a doctor. She has been asking for her mother to be seen by a psychiatrist for over three months, and is upset that her mother's mental health has only now been taken seriously. You should meet with her to address her concerns. You will also be expected to discuss treatment with her.

Suggested points to cover:

1. Allow daughter time to express her frustration.

2. Acknowledge her concerns.

3. Suggest ways in which mental health services may help her mother.

4A A 38-year-old woman with a diagnosis of schizoaffective disorder has asked to meet with you. She has had four previous inpatient admissions and takes lithium and olanzapine. She is in a relationship with someone who has schizophrenia. They want to have a baby together and she would like to know what is the risk of the baby developing a mental illness. She is also worried about the risk of taking medication during pregnancy. You should meet with the patient to discuss the genetic cause of schizophreniform illnesses and the risks associated with taking psychotropic medication during pregnancy.

Suggested points to cover:

1. Explains risks vs. benefits.

2. Discuss likelihood of foetal abnormality.

3. Discuss likelihood of child getting schizophrenia.

4B Since you saw the patient, she has become pregnant. You have been asked to speak with her GP who wants to know more about schizoaffective disorder. She is concerned that childbirth can make mental illnesses worse and would like to know what steps might be taken to manage this risk. You should speak to the GP and address her questions.

Suggested points to cover:

1. Explain risk of becoming unwell and precautions.

2. Discuss symptoms to monitor for.

3. Explain treatment options if becomes unwell.

Individual stations

1 You are asked to assess Steve, a 25-year-old man at your clinic. He tells you he wants to 'turn his life around' and stop using illicit substances or his boyfriend will leave him. Take a history of his poly drug use and assess if he is substance dependent.

Suggested points to cover:

1. Assess details of drug use e.g. what, amount, when.

2. Assess dependence e.g. compulsion, poor control, withdrawal, tolerance, primacy, persistence despite harm.

3. Consider motivation to change.

2 You are about to see an 80-year-old woman who believes that her neighbours are trying to spy on her. The community social worker has informed the ward staff that she has covered the floor with aluminium foil, and was keeping the curtains drawn before she was admitted to your ward. Discuss these with her. You do not need to assess her cognition.

Suggested points to cover:

1. Why does she believe her neighbours are trying to spy on her?

2. Why is she covering the floor with foil?

3. Is she experiencing any perceptual disturbances?

3 Carl is a 45-year-old man who has recently commenced on dosulepin for a depressive illness. He is complaining of 'strange sensations'. The GP wants you to rule out temporal lobe epilepsy.

Suggested points to cover:

1. Enquire around the timing of the symptoms.

2. Attempt to establish exact symptoms regarding seizure type.

3. Screen for psychosis.

4 A GP has asked you to see a 52-year-old man who has been complaining of erectile dysfunction. He has requested sildenafil (Viagra) on more than one occasion. He told his GP that he has been unable to have sexual intercourse with his wife, and that he no longer feels like a man. You should address the man's concerns and do a mental state examination. You should assume that all physical causes of erectile dysfunctional have been excluded.

Suggested points to cover:

1. Discuss details of the symptoms.

2. Enquire about partner's attitude.

3. Screen for anxiety and depression.

5 Mr Harris is a 32-year-old man who is currently unemployed. He has obsessive—compulsive disorder (OCD). He has already been through a course of cognitive behavioural therapy (CBT) which focussed on Exposure Response Prevention (ERP). Whilst this has helped, he still has symptoms. The GP has asked you to see him to consider initiating medication. You should address the patient's questions and explain the role of medication.

Suggested points to cover:

1. Explain the role of SSRIs.

2. Explain antidepressants are not just for depression.

3. Explain potential side effects and address concerns.

6 Mr Matthews is a 50-year-old carpenter who has been referred to your outpatient clinic by his GP. He has marital problems, and his wife has threatened to leave him. His son told the GP that he has been accusing his mother of having an affair. This has upset his mother and has caused hostility in the family. The son is worried that his parents may get divorced because he has seen them rowing on several occasions. You should see the patient to assess the risk that he poses to his wife and others.

Suggested points to cover:

1. Elicit evidence of pathological jealousy.

2. Explore thoughts of harm to wife, rival and others.

3. Assess mood.

7 The daughter of a 79-year-old man has asked to meet one of her father's doctors. She has been told that her father has Alzheimer's disease. She has been reading about the condition and wants to find out about 'dementia drugs'. An MMSE was recently carried out in memory clinic and the patient scored 14. Discuss the management of dementia with the daughter. You should also consider other options.

Suggested points to cover:

1. Provide information about dementia medication.

2. Explain the significance of MMSE scores.

3. Discuss other options such as day centres and occupational therapy.

8 A 73-year-old woman has been admitted to one of the elderly care wards after an emergency home visit. The community team found her living in squalid conditions and on admission her hair was matted with faeces. There have been reports that she has been using offensive language and has been acting suspiciously. The nurses have observed her laughing one minute and then crying the next. You have been asked by your consultant to carry out frontal lobe tests. You do not need to assess her overall cognition.

Suggested points to cover:

1. Assess verbal fluency.

2. Assess abstraction.

3. Assess response-inhibition and set-shifting.

MOCK EXAMINATION 3

Paired stations

1A The GP refers a 35-year-old woman with depression to your outpatient clinic. She had an episode of depression a few years ago, which responded well to fluoxetine. She stopped fluoxetine about three years ago. However, six months ago she became depressed again. Her GP restarted her on fluoxetine around this time but she failed to respond. The GP then changed her medication to venlafaxine. In spite of this, the patient remains depressed. The GP would like you to advise on further management. You should discuss management options with the patient.

Suggested points to cover:

1. Explore her life situation and whether it is contributing to her low mood.
2. Elicit symptoms of depressive illness.
3. Discuss augmentation strategies and psychological therapies.

1B It is now six months later. After your assessment it was recommended that the patient's venlafaxine was augmented with lithium therapy. She has been well for three months, and now wishes to start a family. The GP has asked to speak to you to discuss her management during pregnancy. You are about to speak to him on the telephone. You will be expected to discuss the risks associated with taking medication during pregnancy.

Suggested points to cover:

1. Consider whether or not to stop lithium before conception and during the first trimester.
2. Discuss possible risk with lithium (Ebstein's anomaly).
3. Consider changing the antidepressant to one with more evidence in pregnancy.

2A You have been asked to see Carl Jones, a 43-year-old married man. He gives a seven year history of exposing himself in public. He went to see his GP after he read an article on the front page of the local newspaper about a man who was seen flashing in the park. Mr Jones became very frightened and is worried that he may get caught by the police. The park is next to some school playing fields. The GP said there are some marital problems and that his wife has been in a wheelchair for the last eight years. Before speaking to you, Mr Jones wants to know whether your assessment is confidential. You should take a psychosexual history and assess this man's risk.

Suggested points to cover:

1. Explain the limitations of patient confidentiality.
2. Take a psychosexual history focussing on paraphilias and sexual offending.
3. Assess his risk to others including the school children.

2B You are about to discuss this patient with your consultant. You need to be able to discuss the possible risks that this patients poses to himself and others. The consultant wants to know whether you think that the police should be informed.

Suggested points to cover:

1. Explore potential risk to children.
2. Acknowledge obligation to share information if you believe others are at risk.
3. Discuss risk of recidivism and other sexual offending.

3A You are asked to assess a goalkeeper who has been refusing to play since letting in an important goal eight weeks ago. Talk to him to establish what he thinks about this and his reasons for not wanting to play anymore. Focus on any cognitive distortions that may be present.

Suggested points to cover:

1. Consider arbitrary inference and over-generalisation.

2. Consider magnification and minimization.

3. Exclude depressive illness and anxiety states.

3B Talk to his manager about his treatment options and how CBT may help.

Suggested points to cover:

1. Discuss possibility of psychological therapy to address his faulty cognitions.

2. Describe the process of therapy and what this may involve.

3. Inform if depression or excessive anxiety is present, medication may help.

4A You have been asked to speak to the mother of Christopher, a six-year-old boy. She feels that there is something wrong with her child and no-one is listening to her. He has poor communication skills and poor social skills. She tells you he is very different from his brother. Gather further information from her in order to consider the nature of his problems.

Suggested points to cover:

1. Enquire about social interaction.

2. Enquire about communication.

3. Enquire about stereotyped and repetitive behaviour.

4B It is six months later, and Christopher has been diagnosed with an autistic spectrum disorder. He has been receiving additional support at school, and has made some progress. His mother has asked to see you to discuss his diagnosis. She wants to know what else can be done to help her son. You should address her concerns and offer advice about further management and support.

Suggested points to cover:

1. Explain the importance of structured educational programmes and behavioural techniques.

2. Give practical advice and suggest other areas of support e.g. national autistic society and local support groups.

3. Discuss the limited role of medication.

Individual stations

1 Tina is a 36-year-old woman presenting to A&E with restlessness and agitation. She has marked restless type movements of her legs on observation and cannot appear to keep still. She was recently prescribed 'Halo something' by her GP for three days as she had become increasingly worried that people at work were talking about her and could not sleep. Address her concerns.

Suggested points to cover:

1. Establish whether she is psychotic.

2. Explain that she has probably been given haloperidol and how this causes the symptoms described.

3. Explain the management e.g. the restlessness will go away in a few hours when the medication wears off.

2 A 36-year-old man was picked up by the police after he has repeatedly been loitering outside the local army barracks. He has been seen by the police surgeon who has asked you to assess him as she is concerned about his ideas of what is going on inside the barracks. The police surgeon said he is very suspicious and that her assessment of him was very difficult. You should elicit signs of psychosis.

Suggested points to cover:

1. Enquire why he outside the barracks? What does he think is going on in there?

2. Enquire about his worries and assess degree of distress.

3. Screen for other psychotic features e.g. auditory hallucinations.

3 You have been called to see a patient on the surgical admission ward. The patient, who is a 49-year-old woman, was admitted three days ago with abdominal pain. She has been demanding morphine and became angry when the consultant refused to perform a laparotomy. She has previously undergone two laparotomies, and neither revealed any physical disease. During this current admission all of her blood tests and radiological investigations have been normal. The team became concerned when one of the nurses saw her trying to swallow batteries from her personal music player. You should meet with the patient to take a focussed history. She is expecting to see you but is angry that 'they've called a psychiatrist'.

Suggested points to cover:

1. Explores her worries about seeing a psychiatrist.

2. Attempt to find out how life is for her and enquire about her upbringing.

3. Exclude drug and alcohol addiction or misuse.

4 The mother of an 11-year-old boy who takes methylphenidate for the treatment of ADHD has asked to see you. She is concerned about his sleep. She tells you that since he has been taking the medication he has not been sleeping very well. She feels exhausted and wants to know what else could be done to help.

Suggested points to cover:

1. Take a history of the sleep difficulties.

2. Discuss medication options to include modified release formulations and drug holidays.

3. Inform of appropriate avenues of support for the family and discuss psychoeducation.

5 You have been asked to see a 56-year-old man. The GP is concerned about the amount of alcohol he is drinking. The man lost his job six months ago and his wife has now left him. The GP has carried out tests which show advanced liver disease. You are about to meet the patient. You should discuss treatment and the role of harm reduction. You do not need to confirm dependence.

Suggested points to cover:

1. Explain the results of the blood test and potential consequences of continued alcohol use.

2. Discuss costs and benefits to alcohol use .

3. Discuss alcohol intake monitoring, driving issues and use of vitamin supplements.

6 A 23-year-old woman, who thinks the end of the world is coming next month, has just been admitted to hospital as an informal patient. She was seeing the Early Intervention in Psychosis (EIP) team but it was felt that she would benefit from a period of inpatient assessment. She has only been on the ward for four hours and is now asking to leave. She has told the nurses that they cannot keep her 'locked up' as she is not detained. The nurses are worried about allowing her to leave, and have asked you to assess her. You should focus on her risk.

Suggested points to cover:

1. Discuss her intentions; is there anything she is planning to do to prepare for the end of the world?

2. Consider possible risks to harm herself or others?

3. Exclude depression.

7 Mrs Hunter is a 38-year-old married woman who has two children. She has a diagnosis of depression and has been experiencing negative thoughts about herself for several months and believes that she is a bad mother. She feels guilty that she does not get any pleasure from her two children. She has started to believe that she is a bad wife. You have been asked to see her to discuss psychological interventions. You should not discuss medication.

Suggested points to cover:

1. Discuss the role of cognitive behavioural therapy in treating depression.

2. Discuss the relationship between feelings and behaviour.

3. Discuss how negative automatic thoughts may perpetuate problems.

8 A colleague has asked you to assess an elderly woman who was admitted to the medical ward with fever and confusion. She has since been treated for a urinary tract infection. However, she remains disorientated and is having difficulty dressing. Initially the medical team thought that she was delirious but since recovering from the urinary tract infection, she is alert and eating and sleeping well. You should assess her cognition. You do not need to take a history.

Suggested points to cover:

1. Perform all points of MMSE.

2. Phrase questions clearly and appropriately.

3. Score MMSE.

Paired stations

1A You are called to see a 15-year-old girl in A&E who has cut her wrists with a shaving razor. She has a history of taking medication overdoses. She told the A&E officer that she has been getting bullied at school. She does not feel that she has been able to tell anyone how she feels. You should take a history, focussing on the problems she has been having at school. You will need to talk to your consultant about this girl and will need to consider how she can be managed.

Suggested points to cover:

1. Enquire about the bullying to include the exact nature and any precipitants.

2. Enquire about the circumstances of the overdose and current thoughts about this.

3. Exclude depression.

1B You should speak to the consultant to discuss your findings. You will be expected to discuss diagnosis and to formulate a management plan.

Suggested points to cover:

1. Explain the nature of the girl's difficulties.

2. Consider follow up and its location.

3. Discuss the role of the school.

2A A 26-year-old man is referred to you by his GP. The man has a diagnosis of paranoid schizophrenia and receives a depot antipsychotic agent every two weeks. Over the last three months he has developed bilateral gynaecomastia. He is demanding that you stop his medication as he is convinced that it is responsible for the excess breast tissue. You should assess his ongoing need for medication and explore other important side effects.

Suggested points to cover:

1. Enquire about previous psychiatric history, including compliance with oral medication and number and severity of relapses.

2. Assess level of insight.

3. Enquire about other side effects including impotence, stiffness, tremor, expressionless face and weight gain.

2B You are about to meet his mother. She tells you that her son is very distressed by his excess breast tissue. She wants to know whether the medication is to blame for this. As well as addressing her concerns you should gather further information, paying particular attention to the impact that his side effects are having on his social functioning.

Suggested points to cover:

1. Establish exactly what the mother's concerns are?

2. Enquire about the effect on his relationships, e.g. girlfriend's attitude.

3. Enquire about other effects e.g. social interactions, mobility, eating and drinking.

3A You have received a call from the manager of a local care home. She is calling about a 76-year-old male resident who was on your assessment ward 18 months ago. She tells you that he has recently become aggressive and on two occasions has hit out at her staff with his walking stick. You should take a focussed history from the care manager to explore the possible reasons for this recent change.

Suggested points to cover:

1. Ask whether there has been any recent physical illness.

2. Ask whether there have been any recent changes e.g. in staffing or environment.

3. Ask whether the aggression varies throughout the day e.g. 'sun-downing'.

3B It is four weeks later and the patient has been commenced on a small dose of Quetiapine. Since starting the medication, he has been less aggressive. However he still sometimes goes to grab his carers by their uniforms. The patient's wife has asked to see you. She is very upset and embarrassed that her husband has been 'playing the nurses up'. Discuss the situation with the patient's wife.

Suggested points to cover:

1. Allow wife time to express distress.

2. Acknowledge that it must be a difficult time for her.

3. Reassure her that his behaviour is a symptom of his dementia.

4A You have been asked to see Elizabeth, a 17-year-old girl who has been referred to you by her GP. The GP letter states that she has had low self-esteem for several years. There have been times when she has been unable to go to school despite encouragement from her supportive parents. However, it has now emerged that she is worried about getting up in the morning as she is preoccupied with the idea that something bad will happen unless she gets up in a certain way. She told her mother that for the past three years she has had to get up in a series of complicated steps. This ritual has become more and more complex to the extent that she now freezes on waking for over an hour, fearing that she will make a mistake. The GP now believes she has OCD, and after talking to the family, he has convinced them that she needs a psychiatric assessment. You should meet with Elizabeth to confirm the diagnosis.

Suggested points to cover:

1. Take a history of the start of the difficulties.

2. Enquire about the perceived consequences.

3. Thorough exploration into the detail of the rituals and associated thoughts.

4B You are now about to meet Elizabeth's mother, who wants to know whether you think she has got OCD. She tells you that she thought people who had OCD have problems with not knowing when to stop washing their hands. She is worried that Elizabeth's education will suffer and that she will not be able to go to university. You should meet with the mother to discuss your findings and to offer some information about the diagnosis. You should assume that Elizabeth has given you her consent.

Suggested points to cover:

1. Explain that Elizabeth has obsessive compulsive disorder (OCD) and what leads to that diagnosis.

2. Explain what OCD is and what symptoms can be involved.

3. Explain the treatment of OCD including behaviour therapy and SSRI's and the rationale behind them.

Individual stations

1 Jayne is a 30-year-old lady who works as a solicitor. She is getting married in three months and is feeling very anxious about it. She is worried she may have to cancel the wedding. Take a history of her difficulties and focus on aetiological factors.

Suggested points to cover:

1. Enquire about the relationship and marriage e.g. what is the relationship like whose decision was the marriage, view of relatives, her views on marriage.
2. Enquire about anxiety in other situations.
3. Exclude depression.

2 You are about to see a 73-year-old woman who was admitted after being seen in the community by the crisis team. The crisis team was contacted after the GP was called by the patient's son. The GP and the crisis team found her in bed surrounded by unopened tablet packets. She told the team that she is rotting from within and is frightened to drink. The team arranged an urgent admission to the old age psychiatry ward. You should assess her mental state. You do not need to assess her risk.

Suggested points to cover:

1. Elicit delusions of nihilism.
2. Explore why she is frightened to drink.
3. Assess mood.

3 A 23-year-old medical student has been admitted to hospital after his housemates became concerned and contacted his GP. He had been isolating himself and had told them that the dean of the medical school wanted him to fail his exams. Two weeks previously they noticed that he had taped clear film to his window. Since admission he has been started on a low dose of an antipsychotic medication. He has made a good response and the team are planning to discharge him in the next few days. He has asked to see you to discuss his diagnosis, as he is worried that he may have schizophrenia like his mother. You should address his concerns.

Suggested points to cover:

1. Ask him to describe what has been troubling him lately.
2. What form does his mother's illness take? Are his experiences at all like hers? If so, what is particularly worrying him about this?
3. Explain how his illness and treatment might differ.

4 A nurse from one of the inpatient wards has telephoned you to say that one of his patients has just returned from day leave. The patient, who is 34 and has a diagnosis of schizophrenia, has a history of misusing illicit substances. The nurse requested a urine sample from the patient to see whether he had been smoking cannabis, as he had noticed that the patient was acting bizarrely. The patient refused and has now become agitated. You should meet with the patient to discuss urine testing with him.

Suggested points to cover:

1. Ask the patient why he has been acting in an unusual way.
2. Find out why is refusing and say he has the right to refuse a urine test.
3. Explain why want a urine test e.g. we need to know if it is illness or drugs which have been disturbing him.

5 The GP of a nine-year-old boy has telephoned you for advice. She tells you that the boy is still wetting his bed, and sometimes wets himself when he is at school. She is unsure what to do. She has met with the parents on a few occasions but the problem continues. She has ruled out physical causes and wants to know how she should further assess the boy. She also wants to know how she might manage the problem. You should address the GP's concerns and offer appropriate advice.

Suggested points to cover:

1. Enquire about potential precipitants e.g. stress in the family.

2. Discuss behavioural techniques such as toileting after meals and reward system.

3. Reassure that most have a full recovery.

6 You are asked to review Carly, a 19-year-old mother of a four month old baby. Her partner is concerned she is depressed. Assess her mental state. You do not need to perform a risk assessment.

Suggested points to cover:

1. Enquire about the effects of the baby e.g. Is she enjoying the baby? How often does she wake at night and is it only to feed the baby? How exhausted does she feel?

2. Ask about anxiety symptoms.

3. Ask about depressive symptoms including suicidal ideas.

7 Your consultant has decided to start one of your inpatients on lithium. The patient has a diagnosis of bipolar affective disorder. You have been asked to give him advice about lithium treatment and address his concerns. His mother took lithium for over 30 years but stopped after she developed kidney problems. You also know that she rarely received annual blood testing.

Suggested points to cover:

1. Explain the benefits of lithium e.g. very effective.

2. Describe the monitoring process and frequency e.g. lithium levels, kidney and thyroid function tests.

3. Explain the rationale and benefits of regular monitoring.

8 A 42-year-old woman turned up without an appointment to the psychiatric hospital where you work. She said that she feels depressed and desperate. She told the reception staff that she wants to kill herself. The nurse in charge was called and took the woman to the assessment suite. The nurse is very concerned as the patient is complaining of blurred and double vision. The nurse thinks she needs to be transferred to the medical ward for urgent assessment and has asked you to examine her. You should examine her cranial nerves. You do not need to perform fundoscopy and should not attempt to test her corneal and gag reflexes.

Suggested points to cover:

1. Test visual fields and eye movements.

2. Test facial sensation and facial movements.

3. Assess speech, cough and tongue movements.

Paired stations

1A It is 23:00 hours and you are called by the duty senior nurse who tells you that there is an irate man in reception, demanding to see a nurse from Daffodil Ward. The security staff are now with him, and you are asked to talk to him. The man, who is 38 years old and unemployed, said that he needs to see the nurse because they are in love. The duty senior nurse tells you that the nurse in question is not in the hospital, and does not know how he knows her. You should assess his risk.

Suggested points to cover:

1. Ask how he first came to think he was in love with the nurse.

2. Ask what else has he done and what does he intend to do.

3. Assess for psychosis and enquire about substance use.

1B Since speaking to the man, your consultant has been contacted and you have now been asked to telephone him at home. You should be able to discuss the risk that this man poses in order that you are able to formulate a management plan.

Suggested points to cover:

1. Decide whether or not you think the nurse is in danger from him and if so that she must be told, whether or not he gives permission.

2. If he is not considered immediately dangerous he can be allowed to go home and seen at an early outpatient appointment.

3. Consider use of the Mental Health Act.

2A Mr Roberts is a 60-year-old man, who was admitted to hospital three days ago with a fractured neck of femur and a Colles' fracture. He sustained these injuries after falling down the stairs at home. The orthopaedic nurses tell you that he is acting bizarrely and appears confused. They have also noticed that he 'makes thing up' like what he has eaten for breakfast, and yesterday he told one of the surgeons that he had just been on the bus despite the fact that he is bed-bound. On admission there was a strong odour of alcohol and his speech was slurred. You should take a focussed history and perform a brief cognitive examination.

Suggested points to cover:

1. Enquire about his current difficulties.

2. Assess orientation.

3. Assess short term and concentration.

2B You are about to see the nurse in charge. The nurse tells you that he keeps trying to get out of bed and the nurses are worried about him putting weight on his hip. So far they have managed to stop him, but now they are forced to use rails on the side of his bed, which he has been rattling at night. The other patients have complained that this has been keeping them awake. You should meet with the nurse to discuss your findings with her. You should be able to offer management advice.

Suggested points to cover:

1. Explain the likely cause of his difficulties e.g. alcohol.

2. Explain treatment options including use of pabrinex and benzodiazepines.

3. Offer further education and support for staff.

3A You have received a referral to see a 19-year-old man who was admitted to the medical ward with hypokalaemia. He has a BMI of 16. He was previously known to child and adolescent mental health services, which had concerns about his eating pattern. You should take a focussed history to consider the diagnosis of an eating disorder.

Suggested points to cover:

1. Enquire about eating pattern in detail.

2. Take a history of the how it began, how long it has been going on, family attitude, CAMHs input.

3. Assess insight.

3B After meeting with the patient, you have been asked to go and speak to the nurse in charge. The nurse is worried about the patient because she knows that his heart could be at risk if he does not maintain adequate potassium levels. She tells you that he has been commenced on potassium supplements but is concerned that he will not take them. She thinks he should be admitted to your ward. You should discuss your findings and address her fears and concerns.

Suggested points to cover:

1. Agree with the nurse that it is difficult for her to have patients with psychological problems on a medical ward, but say that as long as there is concern about his physical state, that is the best place for him.

2. Suggest that the dietician is involved.

3. Say you will take over his care when his physical condition is safe enough and offer support in the mean time.

4A You are asked to see a 43-year-old woman who has a diagnosis of borderline personality disorder. She was admitted to the general hospital three days ago after she cut her left wrist. She has had over 15 admissions to the mental health unit and she wants to be admitted again. Before you see her, the duty senior nurse asks you to carefully consider the risks and benefits before agreeing to a further admission. He wants you to contact him as soon as you have seen the patient to discuss your management plan. You should assess the risk she poses to herself and others. You should not agree to an admission until you have consulted the senior nurse.

Suggested points to cover:

1. Enquire about the circumstances of this attempt and any previous attempts.

2. Ask if she intending to harm anyone else or has done in the past.

3. Explore her reasons for wanting admission.

4B You are about to see the senior nurse. He shows you a management plan that was written by the patient's consultant, her care coordinator and the psychologist who she has been seeing for dialectical behavioural therapy (DBT). The plan states that the patient should only be offered an admission if her risk is immediately life-threatening. Discuss possible admission in light of this.

Suggested points to cover:

1. If the risk is not immediately life-threatening she should be told that she is to go home and she can see a member of the community team the next day.

2. Explain admission will be time limited and may not be helpful.

3. Explain what may be beneficial e.g. DBT.

Individual stations

1 One of the community nurses in the child and adolescent mental health service has received a referral to see an 11 year-old-girl who has been refusing to go to school. Her parents are really concerned about her, and despite their best efforts to get her to go to school, she refuses to. When her parents demand that she goes to school, she locks herself in the bathroom until they promise her she can stay at home. The community nurse has made an initial assessment, but is worried that she may be depressed. You should meet with the mother to take a focussed history and to address her questions about treatment.

Suggested points to cover:

1. Enquire about precipitating factors and current life stresses.

2. Assess for depression.

3. Assess for anxiety.

2 You have been asked to see Robert James, a 36-year-old coach driver. He was recently involved a road traffic accident whilst driving a group of children and their teachers to France on a school holiday. Since the accident, he has had problems sleeping and has been unable to work. You should take a focussed history, paying particular attention to the problems he has been experiencing since the accident.

Suggested points to cover:

1. Enquire about symptoms of post-traumatic stress disorder, including flashbacks, bad dreams, numbness and avoidance of reminders of the accident.

2. Ask for symptoms of anxiety and depressive illness.

3. Ask about suicidal ideas.

3 Mr Singh is a young teacher who has been complaining of low mood and low self-esteem for several months. Initially the GP referred him for CBT in the local community mental health team. Whilst he found this useful, he has now developed problems sleeping, a poor appetite and has been complaining that he no longer enjoys anything. The GP has suggested antidepressants but the patient is reluctant to take medication. The GP would like your advice. You should see the patient and elicit symptoms of depression. You should also discuss the issue of medication.

Suggested points to cover:

1. Ask about the depressive symptoms. Enquire how he copes with such a demanding job.

2. Explain that a combination of CBT and medication can be better than either alone.

3. Enquire about his reasons for not wanting medication and explain about antidepressant therapy.

4 You are about to see Mrs Smith, the mother of a 19-year-old patient who has a six year history of binge eating and vomiting. Her BMI is 27. She has never told anyone about her eating pattern, but recently her mother noticed sores on the back of her knuckles and some discolouration of her teeth. Eventually the patient told her mother everything, and her mother is very upset. The GP diagnosed bulimia nervosa and you have been asked to meet with Mrs Smith to address her fears and concerns. You should also discuss treatment options.

Suggested points to cover:

1. Explain that though unpleasant most people recover with treatment.
2. Explain that seeing a psychologist can be helpful, for cognitive behaviour therapy (CBT), for example.
3. Explain the possible role of antidepressants.

5 You are seeing a patient who is about to be discharged from hospital. The patient, who has schizophrenia, is now stable on risperidone. However, before he was started on this medication he threatened his partner with a knife. His partner is worried that he will do it again. Assess his risk of future violence.

Suggested points to cover:

1. Explore whether he intending to carry out his threat.
2. Explore whether he has a history of violence.
3. Explore whether his actions were driven by psychosis.

6 You are about to meet a 60-year-old woman who believes that she is dead. Her friend found her trying to set fire to her house. Establish the nature of her delusions and find out whether the delusions are primary or secondary.

Suggested points to cover:

1. Ask why does she think she is dead and how sure is she of this.
2. Assess if the delusion is completely impossible to understand..
3. Assess mood and physical health factors.

7 A 38-year-old woman with schizophrenia, who has had several previous inpatient admissions, continues to experience distressing hallucinations and believes that her body is controlled by her sister. She has tried several antipsychotics including haloperidol, olanzapine and risperidone. The consultant would like you to discuss clozapine treatment with her. You should assume that she has had adequate trials of the other three medications.

Suggested points to cover:

1. Explain the benefits of clozapine e.g. it is the best drug for schizophrenia where other treatments have not worked well enough.
2. Explain the potential risks of clozapine including serious harmful effects on white cells in the blood.
3. Explain the process of commencing clozapine and the necessary monitoring.

8 Mr Thomas is a 48-year-old man with schizophrenia. He has been stable on an antipsychotic for several years but has recently become unwell. During his admission you diagnosed type II diabetes mellitus. Your consultant has asked you to perform ophthalmoscopy and to discuss the findings with her.

Suggested points to cover:

1. Position patient appropriately and assess red reflex.
2. Assess each eye in turn systematically including the macula.
3. Discuss the findings of diabetic retinopathy.

MOCK EXAMINATION 6

Paired stations

1A You are about to see Mr Young, a retired farmer. His GP is concerned because he has not been sleeping for two weeks. There is some suggestion that he has been irritable, verbally aggressive towards his neighbour and has been talking about 'becoming a multi millionaire'. Take a history.

Suggested points to cover:

1. Ask why he thinks he is a millionaire?
2. Take a history of manic symptoms, now and in the past.
3. Take a history of depressive symptoms, now and in the past.

1B You are about to meet Mr Young's wife. You should discuss diagnosis and management of what you believe to be a manic episode.

Suggested points to cover:

1. Explain bipolar disorder and why you think Mr Young has it.
2. Discuss possible medications, including mood stabilizers.
3. If the episode is severe he may need an in-patient admission, and if milder, he will need follow up by at least one member of the psychiatric team.

2A You are about to meet a 14-year-old boy in the child and adolescent outpatient clinic. The boy has two convictions for stealing cars, and was cautioned last year for threatening to stab one of his teachers. He has a history of shoplifting and taking money from his mother's purse. His mother told the GP that she is worried that he has been bullying his two younger brothers, after his youngest brother tried to run away from home. The boy is reluctant to see you. You should meet with him to take a history. You should also consider possible diagnoses. You do not need to take a detailed risk history.

Suggested points to cover:

1. Enquire about the timing of the problems and any precipitants.
2. Enquire about school and how he gets on with others.
3. Enquire about law breaking and antisocial behaviour.

2B Your consultant wishes to speak to you about the boy you have just seen. She wants to know the differential diagnoses and wishes you to formulate a management plan.

Suggested points to cover:

1. Consider the diagnosis of conduct disorder.
2. Discuss the option of family therapy.
3. Discuss the role of parent training and education programmes.

3A You are about to see a 40-year-man who was last seen in outpatient clinic six months ago. He has a diagnosis of recurrent depressive disorder. He is currently taking fluoxetine. Whilst his mood has greatly improved, he is unwilling to continue taking it. You should explore the reasons for his reluctance to take his medication. His wife is waiting outside, and has asked to meet with you afterwards.

Suggested points to cover:

1. Ask his reasons for wanting to stop fluoxetine.

2. Enquire about side effects.

3. Take a history of previous antidepressant use and what happened when he was off all medication.

3B After speaking to the patient, you have invited his wife to join you. However, the patient has asked to leave. She is frustrated about the situation and demands that you change his medication. You should assume that the patient has given you his consent to talk to his wife. You should address her fears and concerns.

Suggested points to cover:

1. Assess her worries that he will relapse again.

2. Say you will review his previous medication and see if there is a good alternative to fluoxetine for him.

3. Explain that ultimately it is the patient's decision, whether or not to take medication.

4A May is a 48-year-old woman with a depressive illness. She has been seen in your outpatient clinic every month for the last six months. She has been tried on several different classes of antidepressants including selective serotonin reuptake inhibitors, tricyclics and related antidepressants. Discuss further management options for her treatment resistant depression.

Suggested points to cover:

1. Discuss the possible addition of lithium.

2. Discuss the possible addition of a low dose antipsychotic.

3. Discuss the possible use of ECT.

4B May was started on phenelzine and several days later, you receive an urgent call from the ward. She has been complaining of a throbbing headache. The nurses have taken her blood pressure and were alarmed to read a value of 210/95. Her blood pressure is usually normal. When you arrive on the ward you find out the patient has just collapsed. She is not breathing. The ward is in a separate mental health unit and the nurse in charge has gone to call an emergency ambulance. You should provide basic life support until she returns. You will be told when to stop basic life support and will then be expected to provide information to the paramedic. You should address the resuscitation dummy as if it were the patient.

Suggested points to cover:

1. Check and open the airway with chin lift, assess breathing and pulse.

2. Perform rescue breaths and chest compressions at a ratio of 30:2.

3. Stop when paramedics arrive, inform of phenelzine medication and state possible diagnosis of MAOI hypertensive crisis.

Individual stations

1 One of the carers at a group home for people with learning disabilities has asked to see you. She is concerned about James, a 51-year-old man with Down's syndrome. She said that he is having trouble dressing himself and sometimes seems lost when they go out shopping. You should take a history from the carer to consider the underlying cause for the problems.

Suggested points to cover:

1. Enquire about James' usual level of functioning.

2. Enquire about current difficulties to include memory problems.

3. Explain the possibility of Alzheimer's Disease.

2 A 27-year-old secretary has just been assessed in A&E after she turned up there requesting protection. She said she was being monitored and her letters intercepted. Meet with her and carry out a focussed mental state examination to elicit symptoms of psychosis.

Suggested points to cover:

1. Ask about the monitoring and how she has come to believe this.

2. Enquire if the is anything else unusual happening and about auditory hallucinations.

3. Enquire about thoughts interference.

3 A 31-year-old shop assistant has been referred to you by her GP. She has a six month history of feeling exhausted. She is worried about losing her job, as she has had to leave the till after only two hours on several occasions and her manager has become annoyed at having to arrange cover. She has been having lots of tension headaches and despite sleeping for up to 14 hours a day she still complains of exhaustion. Physical causes for her symptoms have been excluded. Take a focussed history.

Suggested points to cover:

1. Enquire why she could be feeling like this e.g. any recent life changes.

2. Exclude a depressive illness.

3. Enquire about previous management including medication.

4 A 30-year-old woman is referred to see you by her GP. She was treated with fluoxetine for an episode of depression two years ago. She responded well and is still taking the medication. She now wants to start a family and is thinking of stopping the medication. The GP wants your advice because he is worried that if she stops the medication she may become depressed again. Speak to the patient to discuss her options and to answer her questions.

Suggested points to cover:

1. Discuss the balance of risks to foetus and mother.

2. Take a history of previous episodes of depression and what happened when she stopped the medication.

3. Discuss potential drugs to use e.g. fluoxetine or tricyclics.

5 In your weekly consultant supervision, you are asked to talk your consultant through an ECG of one of your inpatients. The patient is taking quetiapine, and there have been concerns about the QTc interval. You will not be required to calculate this value as it will be given to you inside the station. You should also be able to answer your consultant's questions and consider whether the ECG would affect your choice of medication.

Suggested points to cover:

1. Assess the ECG to include rate, rhythm, axis, p waves, t waves, QRS complex and QT interval.

2. Ask for QT interval corrected for heart rate (QTc), state that this is prolonged and quetiapine is a potential cause.

3. State that you would consider an antipsychotic with less effect on the QTc interval.

6 You have been referred a 67-year-old man who was widowed over six months ago. His daughter has noticed that he has been isolating himself and has been telephoning her to say that he has been hearing her mother's voice asking him to join her. His daughter is concerned about his welfare. You should meet with the patient to explore these concerns and to consider the risk he poses to himself.

Suggested points to cover:

1. Explore his experience of hearing his dead wife's voice.

2. Does he think that he must kill himself to join her?

3. Does he have any plans about killing himself?

7 A 29-year-old woman with a recurrent depressive illness is referred to your outpatient clinic. She has been taking an SSRI medication for over ten years. Whilst she is stable at present, she constantly finds herself in family situations which cause her stress and anxiety. She has been interested in receiving psychotherapy for some time. She has heard of cognitive analytic therapy (CAT) and has asked her GP to refer her for this. You have been asked to meet her to discuss how the therapy works and to assess her suitability for the therapy.

Suggested points to cover:

1. Explore why she wants to pursue cognitive analytic therapy.

2. Explain what happens during cognitive analytic therapy.

3. Discuss how past experiences and feelings affect the way people interact with others.

8 You are about to meet Clive, who is a 50-year-old man attending your clinic at his wife's request. He says she has threatened to leave him if he doesn't stop drinking alcohol. Take a history to ascertain the extent of the problem.

Suggested points to cover:

1. Assess for dependence.

2. Assess effect on his social functioning and employment.

3. Assess the effect on his physical health and relationship.

MOCK EXAMINATION 7

Paired stations

1A A GP has referred a 28-year-old man to your outpatient clinic. He was involved in a fight outside a nightclub two years ago and sustained a head injury. Since then, his mother has noticed a change in his personality. He used to work as a fitness instructor, but lost his job after the members complained that he had made inappropriate remarks about their weight. In the referral letter, the GP said that his mother is finding it difficult to cope after she found him masturbating in the sitting room. You have been asked to meet with his mother to collect a collateral history. You should focus on the changes in his personality since the head injury.

Suggested points to cover:

1. Ask about changes in his behaviour e.g. emotional lability or impulsiveness.
2. Ask about loss of empathy or ability to infer the mental state of others and inability.to plan complex tasks.
3. Ask about apathy, loss of interest in hobbies, family members and finances.

1B You are now about to meet the patient. You should perform a cognitive examination based on your findings.

Suggested points to cover:

1. Assess verbal fluency.
2. Assess abstraction.
3. Assess response-inhibition and set-shifting.

2A You are about to see Bill, a 64-year-old man who has come to see you at the request of his neighbour. The neighbour said she would call the police if he did not. He is believed to have exposed himself to the neighbour and is now at A&E.

Suggested points to cover:

1. Explore why he exposed himself.
2. Assess if he has a history of exhibitionism or other sexual offending.
3. Assess his risk to others.

2B Talk to Bill's wife. She has some concerns around his behaviour towards their granddaughters ad thinks he may have exposed himself to them. Assess his risk.

Suggested points to cover:

1. Acknowledge obligation to share information if you believe others are at risk.
2. What evidence does she have that he has exposed himself to their granddaughters?
3. Ask if apart from the exposure, has he ever abused the children in other ways.

3A The mother of a nine-year-old boy comes to see you in outpatient clinic. Her son has been having problems at school and she has been called in to discuss this. She has been having similar problems at home, and admits that she was quite relieved when she found out that he was the same with his teachers. She said that his biggest problem is that he will not listen and seems unable to do as he is told. His mother has two younger children and is having difficulty coping. Her husband is in the army and she has no other family. You should take a focussed history from her to consider the nature of his problems.

Suggested points to cover:

1. Assess for hyperactivity.

2. Assess for impulsivity.

3. Assess for inattention.

3B It is over two months since you saw the boy's mother. Since then his father has returned from service and has asked to meet with you to discuss his son. His wife told him that you diagnosed ADHD. He tells you that he has never heard of ADHD and wants to know whether he will 'grow out of it'. You should meet with the father to address his fears and concerns.

Suggested points to cover:

1. Explain what is meant by ADHD.

2. Explain the three areas of difficulties and prognosis.

3. Explain the role of medication and behavioural techniques.

4A You have been asked to see a 34-year-old piano teacher on the medical admission ward. She was admitted three days ago after taking a large overdose of paracetamol. The nurse in charge tells you that the patient has no family. She gave her next of kin as a friend who lives 50 miles away. The medical team said that she is medically fit for discharge. You should meet with her to take a history of the overdose and to explore the details of her social history.

Suggested points to cover:

1. Assess circumstances around the attempt e.g. where, how.

2. Ask about relationships and social situation.

3. Assess her feelings about the overdose and exclude depression.

4B You have discussed the case with your consultant and you have agreed to contact the patient's friend. You should assume that the patient has given you her consent. You should discuss your assessment with her and address her fears and concerns.

Suggested points to cover:

1. Ask about the relationship between these two people and what the friend already knows.

2. Ask what support the friend could provide and suggest what she could do to help.

3. Explain what the management plan is for the patient.

Individual stations

1 One of the community nurses asks you to speak to the father of a 23-year-old man who has a moderate learning disability. The man, who lives with his parents, has recently become increasingly agitated at home. He has been smearing faeces and has been hitting himself in the face. His father does not know what to do. You should take a history from the father to consider the underlying cause for the problems.

Suggested points to cover:

1. Take a history of the timing of the difficulties to include any potential precipitants such as recent events or stress in the family.

2. Consider environmental factors such as temperature, situational factors such as boredom and sensory difficulties such as hearing or visual problems.

3. Consider physical health problems and possibility of pain.

2 A 58-year-old woman attends your outpatient clinic. She has been extensively investigated in hospital for breathlessness but no physical cause has been found. They have referred her to you for help with a possible psychiatric cause. Take a brief history to establish diagnosis and explain hyperventilation to her.

Suggested points to cover:

1. Enquire about the details of the attacks e.g. symptoms, duration, precipitants.

2. Explain the process of hyperventilation i.e. that when people panic they breathe faster, this causes them to breathe out too much carbon dioxide and the acidity level of the blood changes, this can cause the person to feel dizzy and get sensations such as pins and needles in their fingers.

3. Explain these attacks are very unpleasant but not dangerous and offer suggestions such as breathing into a paper bag or cupped hands.

3 The mother of a 20-year-old man has asked to see you. Her son has just been diagnosed with schizophrenia. She is upset and wants to know what will happen to her son. The patient is currently on the psychiatric intensive care unit. You should talk to her and address her concerns.

Suggested points to cover:

1. Explain that on the ward he can be given some medication which will help him feel better and behave more normally.

2. Explain that he may be in the hospital for several weeks, but probably not all of it on the intensive care ward.

3. Explain that most people do well on the medication but after discharge he will need to see the doctors and psychiatric staff for follow-up in the community.

4 You are about to see the mother of a 17-year-old girl who has been diagnosed with anorexia nervosa. Her mother wants to know what she can do to help. She is a single mother and is worried that she and her ex-husband are responsible for the patient developing anorexia nervosa. She also wants to know whether her other two children will 'get it'. You do not need to take a history and you should assume that the patient has given her consent for you to discuss her care with her mother.

Suggested points to cover:

1. Explain that there is a slightly increased risk of siblings getting it, but this is rare.

2. Suggest that family therapy can be helpful for the whole family, not just the affected girl.

3. Explain that most patients are treated as out-patients, and only occasional ones need an inpatient admission. Suggest support groups, local organisations and internet sites.

5 You are asked to assess Anka, a 27-year-old lady who moved here from Poland three years ago. She has suffering from chronic pain in her back, although no physical cause can be found. Take a social history and a history of the pain. You do not need to explain diagnosis or management.

Suggested points to cover:

1. Take a history of the pain symptoms e.g. when did it start, what is it like, how often does she get it, what brings it on, what has she found useful.

2. Ask how she finds living in England and what support she has.

3. Enquire about possible financial or accommodation problems.

6 You are working with the liaison team. You have been asked to assess a 43-year-old woman, who was admitted two days ago after taking an overdose of citalopram and paracetamol. She is medically fit for discharge but her doctors are worried that if they let her go, she might take a further overdose. You should see her to explore her risk.

Suggested points to cover:

1. Assess the circumstances of the overdose e.g. where, when, how, how much did she plan it, did she seek help?

2. Assess her attitude to the overdose she took e.g. is she glad she recovered, would she harm herself again?

3. Enquire about previous self harm and exclude depression.

7 You have been asked to see Sarah, who is well known to your team. She has a diagnosis of borderline personality disorder. She has had trouble controlling her anger and is constantly fearful that everyone will abandon her. She often copes by cutting herself and has required medical attention on many occasions. She feels empty and alone. Her community psychiatric nurse has suggested psychological therapy. The patient has been reading about 'talking therapy' and would like to know more about it. Discuss the role of psychological therapy.

Suggested points to cover:

1. What does she understand about 'talking therapy'?

2. Discuss the role of psychotherapy in personality disorder.

3. Explain dialectical behavioural therapy.

8 You are seeing an 81-year-old woman on the ward. She has not been coping at home. An MRI scan shows small-vessel disease and evidence of an ischaemic region in the left parietal area, probably an old cerebrovascular accident. As part of your cognitive assessment, you wish to consider her parietal lobe function. You should assess her parietal lobe function. You do not need to perform a full cognitive assessment.

Suggested points to cover:

1. Screen for constructional apraxia by asking to copy drawing.

2. Screen for dyscalculia by asking patient to add four and seven.

3. Screen for astereognosia by asking patient to identify object in palm with eyes closed.

Paired stations

1A You are about to meet a young man with a mild learning disability who has been indecently exposing himself recently. He has a previous conviction for this. His partner, who also has a mild learning disability, is six months pregnant. Social services want to take the baby into care. Address his concerns and give him advice about where he might find help.

Suggested points to cover:

1. Enquire about what he believes will happen and his feelings about this.
2. Enquire about the indecent exposure including any underlying sexual motives.
3. Explain that he can get legal help and advice and what this would entail.

1B You are about to meet the man's mother. She is angry that he has been allowed to father a baby as he 'cannot look after himself'. You should address her concerns.

Suggested points to cover:

1. Give her time to express her anger and agree that it must be difficult for her.
2. Find out what she wants to do about the situation.
3. Explain what is likely to happen to the child and that ongoing support will be provided to her family.

2A You have been asked to visit an 89-year-old woman at her home. She believes that there are people stealing her food. She has seen people walking through walls and told her daughter that she sees brightly coloured circles and squares on the floor. You should explore the nature of her experiences. You do not need to perform a physical examination. She does not have any past medical or psychiatric history.

Suggested points to cover:

1. Explore persecutory beliefs.
2. Elicit partition delusions.
3. Clarify whether visual disturbance represents hallucinations or illusions.

2B You are about to meet the patient's daughter. She lives two streets away and sees her mother daily. There is also a lady who visits twice per week to do light household tasks, such as changing the bed. You should meet with the daughter to gather further information from her. Address her concerns.

Suggested points to cover:

1. Take a history of recent events.
2. Find out whether the daughter believes her mother is coping.
3. Is her mother eating and drinking?

3A You have been asked to see Mrs Johnson, a 50-year-old woman who has been having difficulties leaving her house because of anxiety. She tells you it has happened since she had an episode of feeling breathless and faint in a shop about six months ago. Talk to her to establish the reasons for this.

Suggested points to cover:

1. Take details of the episode to include precipitants and symptoms experienced.

2. Take a medication and substance use history.

3. Exclude depression.

3B You are now about to meet Mrs Johnson's husband who has been very worried about his wife. He is annoyed at the current situation. He wants to know how you might be able to help her.

Suggested points to cover:

1. Acknowledge that it must be difficult for him and enquire about the impact on him.

2. Explain graded exposure and that a psychologist or community psychiatric nurse can support.

3. Explain the role of antidepressants.

4A You are asked to see a 20-year-old student who has developed sudden loss of vision after receiving poor exam results. As well as loss of vision, he has been complaining of double vision. You should take a focussed history, and perform a relevant physical examination. An ophthalmoscope and a red hat pin are available for your use.

Suggested points to cover:

1. Enquire about the onset of the difficulties and associated thoughts and feelings.

2. Perform ophthalmoscopy on both eyes.

3. Attempt visual fields, eye movements and visual acuity.

4B The father of the man you have just assessed has been waiting anxiously outside. He is very worried about his son and is shaking. He is desperate to know what is wrong with his son and what will happen next. You should meet with him to discuss his concerns.

Suggested points to cover:

1. State that he must be very worried but say that it seems to be a reaction to the stress of the exam results.

2. Enquire about the significance of the results for the son and his family.

3. Say that these things usually resolve, and that he will be given some psychological support meanwhile, to help.

Individual stations

1 Mrs Jones is a 41-year-old woman who has been to see her GP complaining of problems with alcohol. She feels that she is out of control and wishes to stop drinking. Her GP has asked you to see her. Assess her motivation for stopping drinking.

Suggested points to cover:

1. Find out her reasons for wanting to stop, any previous attempts and what she thinks will happen this time.

2. Find out what preparations she has made in order to stop drinking, when exactly she plans to do this.

3. Find out if she plans to engage in any post detoxification programmes such as AA and what other support she will have around her.

2 You have been asked by your consultant to carry out a physical examination on a 51-year-old patient who is alcohol dependent. Your examination should focus on eliciting the signs of alcoholic liver disease. You should not attempt to examine for testicular atrophy.

Suggested points to cover:

1. Appropriately exposure the patient and inspect the hands, eyes, head, thorax and legs.

2. Inspect and palpate the abdomen.

3. Test for cerebellar signs, weakness and marked sensory loss.

3 You are working on an intensive care unit. A 27-year-old man has been transferred to you from the courts where he was earlier remanded on bail. He has been charged with actual bodily harm. The nurse in charge is unhappy about the transfer and feels that the man should have been sent to prison. She says that she has to think about her vulnerable female patients and wants to know what you are going to do about it. You should meet with the nurse to discuss the management options.

Suggested points to cover:

1. Acknowledge the nurse's concerns.

2. Explore why the patient was assessed as needing psychiatric admission.

3. Suggest ways of maintaining everyone's safety e.g. nursing observation.

4 You are on call and you have been called to the ward. The nurse in charge tells you that one of the patients, who is under a different team, wants to take his own discharge. The nurse is very concerned because since his admission two days ago, the patient has been restless, has been speaking very quickly and has told everyone about his plans to set up a stock-broking agency in the city. You should see the patient to assess his mental state. You should decide whether you think he is safe to go.

Suggested points to cover:

1. Decide if he a risk to himself or others.

2. Consider assessing under The Mental Health Act.

3. Ascertain level of insight into his illness.

5 You have been asked to see a 27-year-old woman who works as a switchboard operator. She believes that she looks abnormal, specifically that her eyes are too far apart. Assess the nature of her problem.

Suggested points to cover:

1. Take a history of the problems including reasoning behind her views, origins of the problem, certainty of the belief and what she wants to do about it.

2. Exclude depression.

3. Exclude an anxiety disorder.

6 Sandra is a 37-year-old woman who has been having trouble leaving the house. The GP has diagnosed agoraphobia. She used to be able to go out of the house to go food shopping and to fetch her children from school, but over the past six weeks she has been unable to leave the front door. Her husband has accompanied her to your clinic today but she remains highly anxious. Her GP has asked you to consider psychological interventions. Take a history to confirm the diagnosis and discuss the role of desensitisation as part of your management plan.

Suggested points to cover:

1. Take a history of the panic attacks including precipitants, symptoms and associated thoughts and feelings.

2. Explain the process of desensitisation.

3. Explain how she will be supported through this process.

7 You are about to meet Darren who works as a teacher in the local school. He has recently been suspended from his job after he was found burying his pupils' essays in the football field. He tells you that by doing this he will make sure they all get A's in the approaching GCSE exams. He says he knew this after watching the breakfast news about a hurricane in America. Assess his beliefs.

Suggested points to cover:

1. Assess how he came to believe this and his level of certainty.

2. Enquire about other unusual beliefs or anything else odd going on.

3. Enquire about auditory hallucinations.

8 Speak to the mother of a 16-year-old girl who is an inpatient on your ward with anorexia. She has weight loss and hypokaleamia. She has heard that family therapy can help. Address the mother's concerns and explain your management.

Suggested points to cover:

1. Ask mother what she knows about family therapy.

2. Explain how family therapy is thought to help families where a member has an eating disorder.

3. Explain what happens during family therapy.

Paired station

1A Gerald is a 50-year-old man on a medical rehabilitation ward. He has been feeling low since his admission a few weeks ago. He was admitted with chest pain and found to have an acute coronary syndrome and diabetes. Address his concerns.

Suggested points to cover:

1. Enquire about what his physical problems mean to him.

2. Enquire about any other concerns.

3. Screen for depression and suicidal ideation.

1B Discuss his management with the consultant.

Suggested points to cover:

1. Discuss possible medication options.

2. Explain his suicide risk and how that conclusion was reached.

3. Consider a Mental Health Act assessment.

2A You are about to meet Claire. She is 21 and has recently broken up with boyfriend. She has had some difficulties around food in the past and is concerned she may become ill again. Assess her personal and family history with a view to starting psychotherapy.

Suggested points to cover:

1. Take a relationship history.

2. Take a history of the problems with food.

3. Screen for self harm, depression and substance misuse.

2B Discuss with the consultant your potential management plan.

Suggested points to cover:

1. Discuss the possibility of analytic psychotherapy.

2. Consider referral to an eating disorder service.

3. Consider the use of a counsellor at the GP's practice or CBT .

3A You are about to see Paul Matthews, a 48-year-old man who was last seen in outpatient clinic three months ago. Before you see him you receive a call from his social worker to say that he is concerned about the risk Mr Matthews poses to his wife. He has been contacting the community mental health team on a daily basis to report that his wife has 'been at it again'. The social worker tells you that Mr Matthews is convinced that his wife is sleeping with their postman. You also learn that he has a history of violence. You should take a risk history from the patient before discussing the case with the consultant.

Suggested points to cover:

1. Elicit pathological jealousy.

2. Ask whether he has any plans to harm his wife, his perceived rival or others.

3. Explore his history of violence.

3B You have asked Mr Matthews to wait whilst you talk to the consultant. The social worker has already found out that there is a bed on the admission ward. You should be prepared to discuss differential diagnoses and further management.

Suggested points to cover:

1. Provide evidence that he has pathological jealousy.
2. Discuss his risk of violence with reference to his past history and mental state.
3. As well as hospital admission consider other management options such as geographical separation.

4A An urgent crisis assessment has been arranged to take place at the home of a 36-year-old woman who has a history of depression. She has a ten month old baby and is six weeks pregnant. The GP tried to visit her but she refused to see him. Her sister lives five minutes away and she has been staying with her since last week because the patient's husband works long hours. Take a history from the patient and make a brief assessment of her mental state. You do not need to assess her risk.

Suggested points to cover:

1. Assess her subjective and objective mood and diurnal variation.
2. Assess for somatic features.
3. Enquire about her feelings towards the baby.

4B You are now about to see the patient's sister. She is very worried. She wants to know what you are going to do to help. As well as discussing management options, you should address her concerns.

Suggested points to cover:

1. Discuss the use of antidepressants.
2. Discuss the location of the treatment e.g. home versus hospital.
3. Discuss support available e.g. a 'home start' worker, health visitor, midwife, CPN.

Individual stations

1 You are about to meet Leroy, a 19-year-old with a three day history of hearing people talking to each other about him from far away. He thinks it may have something to do with a letter that was sent to his mother from America. Assess his mental state and explore psychopathology.

Suggested points to cover:

1. Explore the specifics and details of the auditory hallucinations.
2. Enquire about thought interference.
3. Screen for substance misuse.

2 One of your medical colleagues has asked you to see an 83-year-old man who was admitted to a care of the elderly ward six weeks ago after he fell at home. The team are concerned about him returning home as he lives alone. He told the nurses that he sees squirrels running up and down the wall and that a little girl sometimes comes to talk to him. He takes co-beneldopa and has diabetes. His visual acuity is good. Assess his mental state. You do not need to perform a full cognitive assessment and you do not need to carry out a neurological examination.

Suggested points to cover:

1. Explore his hallucinatory experiences.

2. Assess orientation in time, place and person.

3. Assess insight.

3 A 30-year-old mother has presented to A&E. She is worried about the thoughts she has been having. She told the A&E officer that she has repetitive thoughts about wanting to scald her five-year-old daughter with water from the kettle. She also becomes worried that she has left the kettle on, and has to check it is unplugged from the socket at least thirty times a day. The A&E officer is worried that she may be hearing voices. You should meet with the patient and assess the nature of her thoughts.

Suggested points to cover:

1. Explore the nature of the thoughts to harm her daughter

2. Find out if there are any other rituals

3. Screen for psychosis.

4 You are about to see Lindsey, a 19-year-old student. She has presented to A&E after taking an overdose. She said that she had no intention of killing herself but did not know what else to do. She does not have any features of depression. This is the fourth time she has presented to A&E and she said the nurses hate her. Take a history and explain that you think she has some personality difficulties.

Suggested points to cover:

1. Enquire about the circumstances of the overdose.

2. Take a relationship history and explore family background.

3. Explain what a personality disorder is, features and possible causes.

5 A 59-year-old lady has been referred by her GP as her husband died four months ago. Assess whether she is displaying a normal or abnormal grief reaction.

Suggested points to cover:

1. Assess what the bereavement has been like for her and what symptoms she has.

2. Screen for abnormal grief symptoms.

3. Explore the pervasiveness of the symptoms and the time course.

6 You have received a telephone call from the ward to ask you to meet with Jill, the partner of a patient who was admitted to hospital several weeks ago. The patient was given intramuscular haloperidol as he required rapid tranquilization. He subsequently developed a high temperature and became rigid. His blood pressure was swinging and he began to sweat profusely. He was transferred to the medical ward where he is being treated for neuroleptic malignant syndrome. His partner is angry that he was given 'such a dangerous drug'. Discuss your management with her and address her fears and concerns.

Suggested points to cover:

1. Agree with her that he is very unwell. Inform that he will get the best possible care and she will be kept informed.

2. Explain the rationale for giving haloperidol.

3. Explain that the reaction he had was very unfortunate and that it is a rare occurrence which could not have been predicted.

7 You have been called to the maternity ward to see a 34-year-old woman who delivered her second child five days previously. Since the birth she has been tearful and has been reluctant to care for her baby. Her husband is concerned because she has told him that she is a bad mother and does not deserve their two children. You should take a focussed history and consider her risks.

Suggested points to cover:

1. Assess her thoughts and feelings about the baby.

2. Assess her risk of self harm.

3. Assess her current mental state and level of support.

8 Your consultant has asked you to see Mrs Peters who is a 48-year-old woman with a long history of depression. She is currently taking venlafaxine and lithium. She was admitted to your ward yesterday after her community psychiatric nurse became concerned that she had not been eating and drinking properly. Since her admission she has been refusing food and drinking hardly any fluids. Your consultant believes that she requires urgent ECT, and has asked you to assess her capacity to consent. You will be required to explain your decision to the patient.

Suggested points to cover:

1. Assess her current mental state and her reasons for not eating and drinking.

2. Assess is she understands what ECT is and why it has been suggested.

3. Assess if she can weight up the information and communicate a decision.

Paired stations

1A You have been asked to see Naomi, a 15-year-old girl who was admitted to the paediatric ward two days ago after taking an overdose of 50 Paracetamol. She has been treated and is now medically fit for discharge. The patient's mother has depression and was admitted to hospital three weeks ago. Her father lives abroad but she has a step-father, who has been looking after her. During your interview, she discloses that she was raped by her step-father. Assess her risk.

Suggested points to cover:

1. Assess factors around the overdose and her current thoughts of self harm.

2. Assess her mood.

3. Give appropriate reassurance regarding the alleged rape, explain what will happen now and do not ask leading questions.

1B You have just received a call to say that there are no child and adolescent beds in the area. You are about to meet the paediatric nurse who has been looking after Naomi. You need to discuss ongoing management and how best to handle her risk. Before you see the nurse she tells you that Naomi's step-father wants to discharge her from hospital.

Suggested points to cover:

1. Explain what Naomi has disclosed and that she is not to be discharged.

2. Advise that a member of staff is assigned to stay with Naomi and that her step father is not to have access to her at present.

3. Explain that child care social services will be informed as soon as possible and will make a further assessment.

2A The father of a 29 man with treatment-resistant schizophrenia has contacted the community team concerned about his son. The patient, is supported by the Assertive Outreach Team. You should gather information from the patient's community psychiatric nurse before speaking to the father. You have also been told that the consultant is considering starting the patient on clozapine.

Suggested points to cover:

1. Get a description of the patient's current symptoms and how much they affect his life.

2. Find out how likely it is that the patient will take oral medication reliably and attend for the frequent blood tests.

3. Discuss the benefits and risks of clozapine and whether it is practical to start it in the community.

2B You are about to speak to the father on the telephone. He is concerned about the amount of alcohol that his son has been drinking. His son often telephones him whilst intoxicated. The father lives over 150 miles away and is only able to visit his son every six weeks. He feels helpless and does not know what to do. He wants his son to be 'put into hospital for a proper assessment'.

Suggested points to cover:

1. Ask why he thinks his son is drinking.

2. Explain that there are alternatives to admission.

3. Explain the role of the assertive outreach team and that they will advise the son about the local alcohol treatment services.

3A A 60-year-old man has presented to A&E. The A&E officer has examined the man and has not found any signs of physical illness. The cognitive examination was normal. However the A&E officer is concerned because the man told him that he believed there to be secret agents in the hospital grounds. The A&E officer therefore would like you to assess the patient. You should explore his beliefs and screen for other psychotic phenomena. You should also assess cognition but should not attempt a full cognitive assessment.

Suggested points to cover:

1. Ask the patient why he thinks there are secret agents in the hospital grounds and what he is going to do about it.

2. Enquire about anything else abnormal going on, does he feel safe, does he hear or see anything when there is no-one around.

3. Ask about personal details e.g. name and address, orientation, age, date and time.

3B You are about to speak to the on call consultant. You have had to ring him at home, and he is eager to establish the nature of the patient's presentation. You will need to consider differential diagnoses and you will need to discuss management options.

Suggested points to cover:

1. Explain that there is no known physical illness and he is cognitively normal.

2. Explain he has a paranoid psychotic illness.

3. Suggest a management plan including consideration of the Mental Health Act.

4A Gemma Stewart is a 33-year-old woman and was admitted to the general hospital with sudden onset paralysis of her right arm and left leg. She has been under the care of the neurologists for the last ten days. Her CT and MRI scans were normal, and her blood investigations were all within normal limits. The nurses have observed that she is able to move the limbs normally whilst asleep, and when the ward doctor lifted her right arm over her face it fell to the side. You should meet with the patient to explore possible psychological causes for her symptoms.

Suggested points to cover:

1. Ask the patient to describe the problem and how it began.

2. Ask about her life and whether she has been under stress recently.

3. Exclude deliberate feigning of symptoms and also psychiatric disorders e.g. schizophrenia and depression.

4B Mrs Stewart's husband has asked to see you. He has been terrified that there is something seriously wrong with his wife. He is worried that the doctors have missed something and tells you that he recently watched a documentary about people who were not taken seriously by doctors, and who went onto get terminal cancer. He is worried that this is what will happen to his wife. You should try to allay his fears, as well as offering some explanation of the cause of her symptoms.

Suggested points to cover:

1. Reassure him that the neurologists are thorough and knowledgeable and various tests they have done have not revealed any serious physical disorder.

2. Explain that there is a very close connection between the body and the mind, and sometimes people suffering severe stress behave in unexpected ways.

3. Explain that if she can move her limbs at night it is likely to be psychological in origin and offer help.

Individual stations

1 You are called by the wife of one of your patients. She tells you that she is at her wit's end as her husband has spent hundreds of pounds on golf clubs and has booked a lavish holiday to the Caribbean. He was last admitted to hospital three years ago and has been maintained on lithium. The patient's wife tells you that he has been flushing his medication down the toilet and has been avoiding his community psychiatric nurse. You should take a focussed history from the wife making sure you address her concerns.

Suggested points to cover:

1. Assess the abnormality of his behaviour; consider duration and severity, medication no-compliance and her opinion on what might help.

2. Enquire about insight and can anyone reason with him.

3. Explain that if his behaviour is abnormal and he will not cooperate with treatment, he may need to be assessed under the Mental Health Act for a hospital admission.

2 You have received a referral from a consultant plastic surgeon who works in your hospital. He wishes you to see Mr Yeung, a 28-year-old man who is requesting a rhinoplasty. The surgeon is concerned that the patient has a mental disorder as he seems to be preoccupied with the size of his nose. You should meet with the patient and assess the nature of his beliefs. You should exclude psychotic phenomena.

Suggested points to cover:

1. Assess how has he reached this conclusion and why.

2. Assess how fixed his belief is.

3. Enquire what others feel about it.

3 The parents of an eight-year-old boy called Tom have asked you to discuss him with his teacher, Miss Jones. She tells you that Tom has difficulties concentrating in class and is always running around. She has tried to control his behaviour but she said that he does not listen to her. She is convinced that Tom has ADHD and wants you to assess him at school. Address her concerns and discuss management options with her.

Suggested points to cover:

1. Enquire about what difficulties Tom has at school.

2. Enquire about any school policy on ADHD and that behavioural programmes can help.

3. Discuss the role of medication and offer further information and support.

4 For the last four months Mrs Green has been complaining of panic attacks. She has been seen by her GP on several occasions. She is fearful that she will have a heart attack every time she feels a pain in her chest. The GP initially gave her some diazepam but is now worried about dependence. He does not know what to do and has asked you to see the patient in your outpatient clinic. You should confirm the underlying diagnosis and address the patient's fears and concerns.

Suggested points to cover:

1. Take a history of the attacks e.g. how did they start, when do they come, what happens, duration.

2. Enquire about specific symptoms e.g. feeling extremely frightened, shortness of breath, a racing heart, pins and needles, feeling faint.

3. Explain that panic attacks are very unpleasant but not fatal. Discuss the role of antidepressants, cognitive behaviour therapy and relaxation techniques.

5 You are about to see a 19-year-old man who has been having difficulties at university. He is afraid of standing up in lectures and has been told that he will have to give a presentation in his history lecture. He is worried that he will vomit in front of everyone and embarrass himself. He has been missing lectures because he sometimes is asked questions, and this makes his heart race. Take a focussed history from him and discuss the diagnosis.

Suggested points to cover:

1. Take a history of his experiences including precipitants.

2. Explain that he is suffering with a social phobia, which is a form of anxiety.

3. Explain potential treatments include CBT and antidepressants.

6 You have been asked to see a 66-year-old man on the old age psychiatry ward who is requesting to change his will. There are some problems within his family and his two sons refuse to be on the ward at the same time. One of his sons has only just found out that he is unwell after being told by a family friend. He had not seen his father for over fifteen years but since finding out about his admission, he has been visiting daily. The nurses are concerned about the patient's capacity to change his will. Address the patient's concerns and assess his testamentary capacity.

Suggested points to cover:

1. Explore reasons for changing will.

2. Apply test of capacity to decision to change will.

3. Ensure that the decision is not driven by psychosis.

7 You are about to see a 32-year-old woman who has bipolar affective disorder in your outpatient clinic. She is stable on a combination on lithium and carbamazepine. She has been smoking since she was 18 years old and now wishes to give up. She wants to discuss ways in which you may be able to help. You should make sure you discuss the role of medication and nicotine replacement therapy with her.

Suggested points to cover:

1. Enquire about her motivation for quitting smoking and discuss if now is a good time.

2. Give practical advice such as date setting, informing those around and discarding smoking paraphernalia.

3. Discuss the role of nicotine replacement therapy and anti-smoking medication.

8 A patient was admitted to the general adult ward yesterday evening. He was found wandering around the train station by the police. He was disorientated and unable to tell the police anything about himself. During the night the nurses observed him having a tonic-clonic seizure and your consultant has now asked you to perform bedside tests of temporal lobe function. You do not need to carry out an assessment of global cognition.

Suggested points to cover:

1. Screen for impaired learning and retention of verbal material by asking patient to repeat an address and recall it three to five minutes later.

2. Screen for anomia by asking patient to name objects such as watch and pen.

3. Assess memory by asking about famous events such as the terrorist attacks on the twin towers.

INDEX

HOW TO PASS THE MCRPSYCH CASC